Watsu

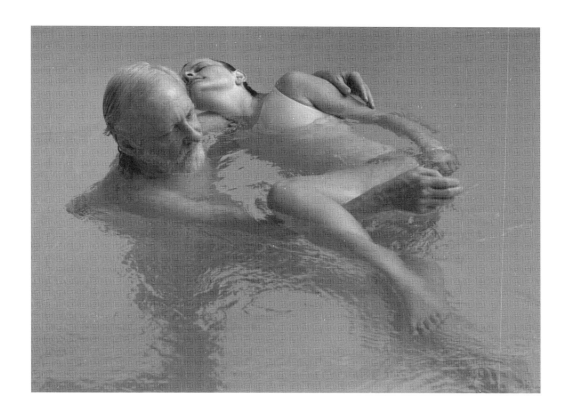

Freeing the Body in Water

by Harold Dull

All the photos of this book, unless otherwise acknowledged, were taken by Bob Ritchie. The assembling of them into movement montages, as well as the design and layout of this book, is the work of the author. Over the years, countless others, here and in Europe, students, colleagues, freinds, have helped in the development of Watsu; most recently, Minakshi, who helped fine tune the sequences as they evolved for this book. Jo Moore gives the Tantsu in the fourth chapter. The author's wife, Valerie, is the lady being floated and stretched all the way through the book.

First edition: April, 1993
LCCC No. 93-77503
ISBN 0-944202-04-7

HARBIN SPRINGS PUBLISHING

Contents

IV WATSU ON LAND

V REBONDING THE BODY

VI EXPANDED FLOW AND VARIATIONS

VII THE REHABILITATIVE BENEFITS OF WATSU

By Lisa Dougherty, Emily Dunlop and Sunny Mehler

VIII DANCING IN THE WATERS *a Woman's Watsu*

by Alma Flor Ada

IX REBONDING THERAPY

X CREATIVE MOVEMENT MEDITATIONS

XI INTIMACY

XII RESOURCES

Foreword

Watsu is on its own

As the final touches go into this book, Watsu is taking hold in Japan. This completes a circle that began when I started applying in water the principles and stretches of the Zen Shiatsu I had studied in Japan. In the ten years it has taken Watsu to find its way back, it has taken root in many countries of Europe. It has been introduced in Canada, in Mexico, in Africa, in Israel, in India, in Australia, in New Zealand . . . and now in Japan. The circle is complete. In completing this book, and the videos that accompany it, much is coming to completion. The problem of how to present Watsu, and make it available to as many people as possible, has been solved with the help of countless students in classes here and abroad. An affordable Watsu pool that can be shipped and set up anywhere has been developed. A new center for Watsu is being built here at Harbin Hot Springs. Watsu has come of age. When I step into Harbin's warm pool and see people I've never seen before watsuing each other, I feel what a parent feels watching a child going out into the world.

No limits

Watsu is as unlimited as the water it is done in. As healing in the giving as in the receiving, Watsu is true co-therapy. There is no limit to the number of people who can benefit from sharing its simplest moves. This is seen in our drop-in classes, and in the wide range of workshops which incorporate Watsu's Water Breath Dance to bring participants closer together. It is seen in aquatic exercise classes which use it as a 'warm down', and in the ease with which groups of children, of pregnant women, of octogenerians learn to Watsu each other. This breadth of Watsu, its reach outward, is matched by its depth, its reach inward. There is no level of our being it can not touch. There is no limit to the ways it can be tailored to individual needs. Physical therapists find it alleviates countless physical and psychological conditions. It has helped the handicapped, the disabled, the depressed, the addicted, the abused, those with aids, hyperactive children, and couples in troubled relationships.

Stages of learning

With this book you learn Watsu in stages that can be spread over as long a period as you want. After an introduction to Watsu, you learn to work with the breath and, in the Transition Flow, to move someone from position to position without interrupting the flow. This simple but powerful sequence has a completeness in itself and can be practiced over and over. After chapters on Tantsu (Watsu on land), and the forms of energy involved, you learn additional moves and detailed bodywork to expand and vary the Transition flow.

Chapters 7 - 12

In the seventh chapter, therapists who work with a variety of conditions at a center for the physically disabled and handicapped present case histories and focus on Watsu's use in rehabilitation. In the eighth, an author of over forty books, sensitively chronicles the effects on her life Watsu has had. This is followed by a chapter on Rebonding Therapy directed to both those who are giving and those who are receiving a series of nurturing bodywork sessions that gradually introduce the non-sexual intimacy our bodies crave but have been denied. The tenth chapter introduces Creative Movement Meditations which can be practiced between sessions. They help you get in touch with the forms of energy, with the freedom and creativity in your body, and can accompany any part of this book. The eleventh explores the nature of intimacy. The final chapter presents resources to aid Watsu's growth and accessibility.

Tapes

The movement meditations are available on video and audio tape. The Transition Flow is available on a videotape, which, besides step by step instruction, presents the sequence in a way which can be followed on land as Tai Chi to practice and internalize the Flow. Seperate videotapes present the Expanded Flow, Free Flow, and Tantsu.

After completing this book I've read Michel Odent's <u>Water and Sexuality</u>, which explores how our sexuality is intimately connected to water. Our uniqueness among primates, our smooth skin, our upright posture, our intelligence, and the way we are drawn to water, are all connected to our ancestors' having passed through a stage as aquatic mammals when the sea rose over much of Africa. Or, as Robert Creeley once said in a poem that begins "Out of the table endlessly rocking..."- "Everything is water if you look long enough."

CHAPTER I

WATSU

It was said in Egypt that water is given the soul as compensation for taking on a bodily form. In water our bodies find the freedom the soul has lost. Watsu is the continuing exploration of that freedom.

Introduction

Warm water is the ideal medium for freeing the body.

Drift and flow

Let yourself be floated and rocked in warm water. Let its total support and warmth penetrate and melt the tension in your body. Drift into deeper and deeper levels of relaxation as your body is stretched freer and freer. Flow into states of consciousness to which stored tension or trauma otherwise deny access. Flow onto a level of Being where there is such joy and peace and wholeness, the causes of that tension or trauma can no longer overwhelm you.

This is Watsu.

And Watsu is as much a joy to give as to receive.

Dance round stillness

Float someone in warm water. Let your body sink as you breathe out and feel how the water lifts you both back up as you breathe in. As your body becomes freer, its movement becomes more and more wave like, waves that rock free the person you hold, as stretch flows into stretch, a slow dance flowing round moments of stillness. Floating someone level with your heart center, there is a connectedness, a oneness that lasts long after a session is finished.

This is the joy of Watsu.

The joy of Watsu

And this joy is as accessible to those first learning Watsu's simplest moves as it is to those who master a full range of techniques. This is seen in our classes here, and in our trainings in Europe. It is something shared by groups of children in Switzerland, and by octogenarians in Italy. When the day comes when the cost of heating pools drops to the point every neighborhood or city block can have its own warm pool where people meet and relax and float each other, it is something that will be available to everybody.

The origins in Zen Shiatsu

Watsu began at Harbin Hot Springs where I came to teach the Zen Shiatsu I had studied in Japan. Zen Shiatsu incorporates stretches which release blockages along our meridians, the channels through which our 'chi' or life force flows. In the orient stretching is an even older therapy than acupuncture which focuses on points along these meridians. It strengthens muscles, and increases flexibility and range of motion. I found these effects can be amplified and made more profound by stretching someone while floating them in warm water. This is corroborated by physical therapists who, working with the handicapped and the physically disabled, find Watsu effects a greater increase in the range of motion than traditional methods. By supporting, rocking and moving the whole body while stretching a leg or arm, Watsu lessens the resistance there is when a limb is worked in isolation. When the whole body is in continual movement, each move flowing gracefully into the next, there is no way to anticipate what's coming next and build up resistance. Without pain, the body can move beyond those limitations fear would otherwise impose. New life is stretched into long neglected connective tissue and the restricted body is shown new possibilities of freedom.

Warm water, and the continuous support it provides, is ideal for freeing the spine. It takes the weight off the vertebrae and relaxes the muscles. Unrestricted by contraction, the circulation can carry away metabolites left over in the muscles, thereby reducing soreness and fatigue. The reduced requirements of oxygen found in states of weightlessness help calm the respiration. The relaxation of tension in the spine and the musculature, by removing excess pressure on the nerves, improves the tone and functioning of the whole body and the organs those nerves service. It allows the spine to be moved in ways impossible on land. This freeing of the spine is so important that it is the focus at the beginning of each Watsu. Even someone not flexible enough to be put into positions for Watsu's more complex stretches, receives great benefits from its simple rocking and gentle gradual twists. And just as stretches and rotations of the arms and legs open up meridians flowing through them, this articulation of the spine helps open its energy pathways. Experiencing this greater flexibility and freedom reprograms a receiver to face life out of the water with greater equanimity and flexibility.

Watsu, as a form of bodywork, is itself flexible. It can be easily learned by people who have had no previous experience in bodywork. Those who have, find it easy to incorporate into Watsu techniques they have learned in massage, deep tissue, Trager, or whatever other forms of bodywork they might have studied. The way Watsu frees and connects giver and receiver facilitates work on that level of intuition and creativity which is the basis of all powerful bodywork.

Watsu affects us on all levels of our being: on the emotional, the psychological, and the spiritual, as well as on the physical. Many of its effects on the emotional are due to the trust Watsu engenders. A person's very life, their connection to the life sustaining breath, is entrusted to the arms of the watsuer. Watsu is the most nurturing of all bodywork. Many get in touch with a sadness at not having been held so before. Some get in touch with feelings locked in parts of their body that Watsu brings back into awareness. Those who get in touch with sexual undertones, have an opportunity to learn, contrary to what they may have been taught, that sexual feelings do not always have to be either acted on or repressed, as they feel them, and whatever other feelings come up, merge into the pleasure their whole body feels being moved through the water. This flow, and the letting go into the flow, is something that can be carried out of the pool long after a Watsu.

Each person is different. What each person gets out of Watsu is different. Some speak of an increasing awareness of where tensions are stored in their bodies, and how to better deal with them. Others overcome a lifelong fear of water. Some float all the way back into the womb. Some re-experience their birth. Many delight at being able to feel the energy coursing throughout their body. And some experience a rising of energy, a moving up into a world of light. Each Watsu is different.

Zen Shiatsu's principle of continuous support takes on a new dimension in water. On land this is furthered through the use of the 'mother hand', the hand that stays in one place while the other hand works. In water, this kind of support, without which the receiver could go under, takes on a new meaning. Once it is realized the support is continual, and trust is established, a powerful bonding takes place, a bonding reminiscent of that between a mother and child . . . or between lovers . . . but one free of any emotional demands or dependency. It is just 'being' with the other. This is the basic principle of Zen Shiatsu- that of Being not Doing. A watsuer comes to each session free of any expectations. We do not try to do something to someone. We do not try to direct them into any particular experience. We do not try to heal them. We just be with them, hold them, support them, float them into whatever they flow into. This profoundly affects receivers who have never experienced anyone being with them this way, in an intimacy as deep as this without any need or intention attached to it. This practice of being with someone profoundly affects the watsuer, and the way they deal with people and life in general. It is as much a spiritual practice as any other form of meditation. To feel the connection one does in Watsu, to feel a oneness with people we would never have imagined any connection, brings home how we are all one. This embodies another principle of Zen Shiatsu- that the person we work with is our teacher.

Carrying the effects out

The effects of giving a Watsu are carried out of the water. In our intensives that combine instruction in water and on land we regularly see how Watsu's freeing of the body, and its sense of connection and flowing movement, carry over into our students' work at a table or on the floor. In our weekend drop-in classes, we see how even a short introduction can give people a new sense of connection with others. Many come back every weekend. Some have told us how giving Watsus has changed their lives, showing them how deep and non threatening an intimacy, a oneness they can feel. Watsu is Rebonding therapy for both giver and receiver.

Differences that challenge

People are different. Some float on top, while those who are all muscle and no fat, sink to the bottom. Besides buoyancy, both size and flexibility effect what a watsuer is able to do. These differences challenge you to be ever more creative, adapting and discovering what works with each person. With some you aren't able to do more than the simplest rocking and stretching (which for those people are as effective as the complex moves you do with others). And with some you find yourselves moving into ever new positions that flow one into the next with a Zen spontaneity. They are the easy ones. The true Zen of Watsu comes when you feel that same freedom with whomever you float around the pool.

Spontaneous as breath

This freedom is as much present in the middle of a sequence as when you are moving someone in Free Flow. This freedom (and love) is being totally present in your own body with the other at every moment. Moving in water is such, that even in Watsu's most basic moves, no two moves can ever be the same. We are always in a new place. The way we move through a sequence can be as spontaneous as our breath, as long as we stay in the moment. The sequence presented in this book has been developed over the years in countless classes here, and in Europe. It is not difficult to learn. It can be done with most people. It moves someone through deeper and deeper levels of surrender and brings them to a sense of completion at the end.

Exploring freedom

Watsu is the exploration of freedom. Feel free at any point to explore on your own, to play. In our sequence you begin with basic moves that you return to again and again. Explore how they vary each time you return. When you learn the transition flow, flowing into and out of the major positions used in Watsu, explore the possibilities each position opens, before going on to see how they are expanded later in this book. Let the slow moving in and out of positions of the transition flow be a model for Free Flow, moving into and out of ever new positions.

Creativity

Watsu is, if anything, creative. It's creativity being attested to by the way those who develop an ongoing practice find their own Watsu. Watsu is so multidimensional and works on so many levels, no two people come at it in exactly the same way. Trying to legislate exactly how it is done and what is supposed to happen, putting a straight jacket on that which is dedicated to freeing the body, would be like trying to tie water with a rope . . . and ending up with a wet knot.

Be with your partner

Be with your partner. Give him or her the space and flow within which to discover the freedom in their own body. Give them the space and flow to move into or out of whatever heart or mind place opens up. However much or however little, welcome it as a gift. Have no expectations. Approach each Watsu as an occasion to practice being with another without expectation.

PREPARATIONS

There are many ways you can prepare yourself to do Watsu. Anything you do to get your own body freer and more centered will be reflected in your Watsu.

In water   Before giving a Watsu, practice the Water Breath Dance described on page 106. Learning to sink and float, and the other practices described there, are also valuable.

On Land   Besides this getting to know water from all sides, there are many practices one can do on land to become more centered and supple such as Tai Chi and Yoga. Continuum, Tantra, and the Movement Meditations all help you become more present to the wave and other movements within your body. Practicing the Co-centering and Tantsu described later in this book helps you become more centered and connected and accepting of others.

Precautions

Never work in water that is over 98° fahrenheit (37° centigrade).

Physical problems   You should not do Watsu with people who have a condition that precludes being in warm water for a period of time. Before a session, familiarize yourself thoroughly with the person and any conditions which might be worsened by pressure or movement. If there are any neck or back problems, find out if there are any movements such as arching the back that might have worsened it in the past and avoid those movements. If, like most such problems, it is related to muscle tension, sensitively applied Watsu can be very beneficial. If, rather, it is a disk problem that any movement will only further aggravate, do not try to watsu the person. Also avoid pressure or excessive movement of any area where inflammation is involved such as a sprain or tendonitis. Be cautious with stretches and rotations with the elderly because of the possibility of their bones being weak and brittle from calcium loss. Avoid pressing varicose veins. Do not watsu someone who has been bedridden for a long time because of the danger of phlebitis. A more detailed list of contraindications appears on page 90.

Limits   Everyone has limits. There are limits to the amount of pressure or stretching they can take, and limits to the degree of closeness or intimacy they can accept. With many, what they perceive as their limit may fall far short of what they are capable. Watsu can help them approach that greater capability by taking them into that unexplored area between their perceived and their actual limits. This cannot be forced. When someone says "This is my limit," that is his limit. We do not try to break through someone's resistance. That can only set up more resistance. Watsu flows them through what were once perceived as limits without creating resistance. The watsuer should be careful not to go beyond their actual limits. The likelihood of this happening is lessened by the slowness with which we move and stretch people. Another reason for maintaining Watsu's slow motion is that many people become dizzy and nauseous if we turn them too fast in the water.

Anxieties   Before beginning determine any problems a person might have with water, or the level of intimacy achieved in Watsu. Watsu can help people overcome any fear they might have around water. Carefully applied it can also be beneficial for people who have problems of trust because of past abuse. It can give them the experience of close nurturing holding, of an intimacy free of sexual intention.

Know your own limits   Be aware of your own limits. Do not try to Watsu someone in water that is too hot for you to work in. Anytime you feel yourself on the verge of overheating bring the Watsu to a conclusion and get out of the water. Do not try to watsu someone who is too big, or too heavy in the water for you. Be aware that in the warm water your muscles might be so relaxed that they may fail to warn you when you are about to strain them. Move out of any position which you feel is on the verge of becoming uncomfortable. Besides being a sign of potential injury, discomfort can keep you from being truly present with the other.

The Neck

The new born

We must take the same care to keep our partner's neck supported as we do with a new born infant. As the muscles in the neck become more relaxed, the danger of hyper-extension, of over compressing the disks and nerves between the vertebrae when the head falls back is increased.

The neck back

Before beginning a Watsu determine how long the person can let their head lie back without discomfort. Even if they can for some time, assume that time may be considerably shortened in Watsu's deeper states of relaxation. Avoid any sudden moves or drops of the head just as you would with a newborn.

Releasing tension

Anytime the head has been back a while during the session, bring it forward to release tension. Pulls of the head can also be beneficial. (Though be aware that pulling the head pulls the spinal cord and can cause pain in the lower back if a nerve is pinched there.) Be specially careful with those who have pain or numbness in an arm associated with pain or stiffness in the neck. This can indicate a pinched nerve in the neck. Keeping the lower back from hyper-extending by supporting under the sacrum and tailbone helps protect the neck, as well as the back.

Supporting the neck

In position one, the position we begin from and continually return to, we support the neck and occiput in the crook of our elbow. Throughout maintain a slight pressure against the occiput to protect the neck. Most people are very comfortable in this position but occasionally there are those who cannot tolerate any pressure against the back of the neck. With them, do as much as possible by holding the head in your hand instead.

You can tell someone to signal any discomfort of the neck during a Watsu by a physical or verbal signal.

The Nose

Keep it out of the water.

Some ride lower

And if it does go under, as just might sometimes happen, keep calm. Some people ride lower in the water than others. When first learning Watsu you can tell the person you will do your best to keep the nose out, but if they happen to feel it perilously close to the surface they should start breathing out of it.

Sometimes it does go under

Without realizing it until the person told me afterwards, once I let someone's nose go under for a moment. I had been aware during the session that she was going through some emotional release. Afterwards she told me that when her nose went under, she recovered a memory of her father trying to teach her to swim, promising he wouldn't let go of her. When her body finally relaxed in the water, he did let go of her and her nose went under. When I let it go under she got in touch with the pain and anger she had repeatedly felt whenever her father betrayed her that way. And though the anger that came up then dissolved in the flow of the Watsu, there was obviously more there than what one could hope to clear in one session. At the end she felt energy streaming out through her whole body. When she told me about it I offered her a chance to get even with me for letting her nose go under. (Though she said she might have done it herself- to get in touch with that event?). I let her push and hold me down under the water. She finally drew me back up to the surface.

The slide to the bottom

Some people, when we let go of them at the end of a Watsu, deliberately let themselves slide down under the water. A final surrender? I had someone do that once when I was demonstrating on several people in Belgium. I didn't realize how long the first one was staying on the bottom until afterwards those around the pool told me how they were beginning to worry about him. It must have been bizarre, watching me lift and stretch the second up out of the water while the first was still lying face up on the bottom. But he finally came up. If you are with someone who drops down to the bottom like that, don't walk away. When people hyper-ventilate, their body may forget to respond to the need for air and may need help up.

But letting yourself slide down to the bottom like that, is completely different from having someone you trust let your nose go under. Don't let it happen. Keep it out of the water.

The Ears

The ear is another story. It's impossible to do a Watsu keeping the ears completely out of the water. Most people who may be apprehensive about the ears going under usually relax and enjoy the feeling and the silence. But some are bothered by the water moving in and out of them. When first putting someone's ears under water leave them completely submerged for three or four minutes.

Ear infections   Some have a tendency toward ear infections. Rinsing the ears afterwards with a combination half alcohol and half white vinegar is a common preventive of swimmer's ear. The alcohol is a drying agent and the vinegar restores the correct PH balance. Ear plugs should be available for those bothered by water entering the ear during a Watsu.

The Pool

Depth   The ideal Watsu pool has many levels so that the practitioner can work with a person at a variety of depths. In a smaller pool with one depth, the depth closest to ideal is about four feet (1.22 meters). In water deeper than this, practitioners can become limited in how wide they can spread their legs, and how much they can use vertical movement. In shallower water, some moves that involve bringing the person to a vertical position become more difficult, but there is a trade off in that in the shallow pool the practitioner can use his legs or knees to support a person.

Size   The larger (and the less crowded) the pool the better. You need enough space to rock and turn with them without their feet touching the wall, at least an eight-foot circle. If you are considering building or installing a pool, check with the school at Harbin. We have available an inexpensive, fully insulated portable pool which is ten feet in diameter. It can be shipped anywhere in the world and set up in less than an hour. It is described on page 119. We are also developing a larger fiberglass pool, as well as a pool that can be fitted onto a pick-up truck for taking Watsu on the road. In addition we are developing plans and specifications for those who want a Watsu compartment in their swimming pool.

Temperature   The ideal water temperature for Watsu is that of the body's surface, about 94° Fahrenheit or 35° centigrade. If the air outside is cold, the water could be a little warmer. If it is hotter than our internal temperature, it is dangerous to work in. When working in warm water, remember to drink copious amounts of water to avoid dehydration.

Music   I prefer to work without background music because its rhythms can mask the inner rhythms our bodies begin to move to in water as they become free.

If you don't have a pool to work in, explore what is available for the handicapped in your community. Many students find volunteering their services at such places to be particularly rewarding.

Individual Differences

Size, flexibility, buoyancy, and holding are parameters that determine how many of the moves included in this book you will be able to do with any single receiver of Watsu. There are people out there whom you might find impossible to watsu. Then there are many with whom, for one reason or another, you have to limit your moves, but who still get a great deal of benefit from what you are able to do with them. Moves you might need to leave out are marked with .

Flexibility   Of the four parameters listed above, you might find flexibility or rather inflexibility the most limiting. Particularly inflexibility that is structural and has to do with shortened tendons, etc. Inflexibility due to holding, may be lessened as the person reaches Watsu's higher levels of relaxation.

Buoyancy   Buoyancy is also important. Some people sink more than others. Muscle tends to sink and fat float. Hence women, who have more subcutaneous fat than men, tend to be better floaters. If you have someone with very developed muscles you probably have a 'sinker' and will need to adapt your positions and how long you can maintain them. The closer you bring someone's center of gravity to your own line of gravity, and the less spread out their weight, the easier they are to support.

Size   If the person is much larger than you, you may have trouble with some moves. But there is still much you can do with the person, particularly if the problem of size is not complicated by problems with flexibility, buoyancy or holding.

Holding   A kind of holding, a holding onto control, occurs when you have someone who wants to do everything for you; someone who, when you start to stretch a leg, pushes it farther. Usually a simple suggestion can help the person surrender. Another area some people try to hold onto control is with their breathing. Some people may force a slow breathing. Others who have had experience with Rebirthing may keep up a rapid breathing which can lead to tetany, a spasmodic tightening of the muscles usually beginning in the hands and mouth, due to hyperventilation. In either case the person can be told to breathe normal deep breaths. The tetany occasionally spontaneously occurs without the person being aware of how they have been breathing. You may need to assure someone unfamiliar with this state, that it, and the tingling sensation that accompanies it, will go away by itself; that it is nothing to worry about.

Not interrupting   Except in circumstances like the above, it is better not to interrupt the process verbally. If you notice tears forming in someone's eyes, or sighing, or some other emotional reaction, it is best to keep holding and floating them, so that whatever is coming up has the opportunity to work itself through in the flow of the Watsu.

On Learning Watsu With This Book

Begin with the easy   Find a warm pool. Go there with a friend who also wants to learn Watsu so that you can exchange roles and feel the moves in your own body. Neither of you should be too big nor inflexible for the other. It is best to first learn Watsu on someone easy to handle and then explore how to adapt to those who present difficulties.

Learn in stages   The sequences in this book, and the order in which they are presented, have been developed and fine tuned in countless classes here and in Europe. In the following chapter you learn to flow from position to position, as you learn the major transitions used in Watsu. Because this transition flow is a continuous flow it is more easily adapted to cooler water than the more detailed Expanded Flow. If you don't have a warm pool to regularly practice in, you can practice this in a swimming pool as long as your partner doesn't become chilled. When the water is cooler than skin temperature (94° f, 35° c). you lose the slower, more deliciously yin side of Watsu. You have to keep moving.. The problem is compounded if the air outside is cold and you have to keep their body always under water. On a summer day, in a not too cold swimming pool, the cool water Watsu transition flow can be an exhilarating experience. And the more you practice it, the more prepared you will be to expand it when you do get to a warmer pool. This flow can also be practiced standing on land with an imaginary partner in your arms, flowing through all the moves as in Tai Chi. A follow-along video tape is available.

In this book the Transition Flow is followed by a basic Tantsu sequence. Tantsu is Watsu on land and it is a good preparation for the expansions. What you learn in the Tantsu about holding points and chakras will make it easier to do the same in the Expanded Flow.

Explore   Once you have mastered the transition flow, explore on your own what possibilities for additional bodywork each position offers. Then learn how each of its three sections are expanded, and a fourth added, in Chapter Six. Practice this thoroughly. Then learn further expansions and variations, a sequence on the steps and the principles of Free Flow.

CHAPTER II

THE TRANSITION FLOW

Flowing from position to position

The Transition Flow is a simple, but complete, Watsu. It incorporates basic moves and the transitions that flow from position to position. Typically there will be one move, rock or stretch that is done on arriving in a position, and another that initiates the flow into the next position. These moves are co-ordinated with the way your body naturally moves in water to the rhythm of your breath. Later in this book, in the Expanded Flow, you will learn additional moves and stretches that can be done in each position.

Beginning with this simple framework makes Watsu easier to learn. It encourages the beginner to focus on how to keep a flow going through a Watsu. It provides a form which has a power and grace in itself, which can be practiced over and over without ever exhausting its potential. Because its flow is continuous, it can be adapted to situations where the water temperature is less than ideal.

Moves and Cradles

After an Opening at the wall, the Flow begins with the Water Breath Dance in which you surrender and free your own body, co-ordinating its movement to your breathing. This slow dance, and the Basic Moves that accompany it, are returned to, are come home to, after each of the three sections that follow. Each section opens with a cradle. A cradle is a position in which you capture or cradle someone between your body and one arm, thereby freeing your other hand to work the rest of their body. If you find when you rotate someone's near leg, that the nearest the knee comes to the chest is a distance greater than the length of your arm, that person is probably not flexible enough to get into a cradle. In this case focus on the Basic Moves and those parts of the transition flow you can do, which can be as effective with someone who is not flexible, as the more complex moves are with someone who is. Moves which may be more difficult than others are marked with an $\otimes$.

Steps to learning

In learning this, begin with the Opening, the Basic Moves and the Completion. Practice these over and over. Then learn the three sections, practicing each thoroughly before going on to the next. Practice the flow over and over until you are able to smoothly flow through the whole sequence with your body's movements effortlessly coordinated to your breathing. The flow can be practiced on land as a form of Tai Chi. Once mastered, explore what opportunities each position offers. Explore how, after completing the third section, you can flow into and out of new positions (Free Flow).

Water Breath Dance

Before starting a Watsu you can get into the pool together and both practice letting go into the water with the Water Breath Dance described on page 106. Carry the feeling of it into your Watsu. Determine if there are any problems with neck, back or any other part of the body that might be worsened by pressure or stretching. Find out if there is discomfort floating with the head hanging back, or if the neck will need continual support (which should be given in any case). Tell your partner to let you know if anything is uncomfortable. If there is a wall that can be leaned against, do the Wall Beginning described below. Otherwise begin standing in the middle of the pool. A third way to begin is possible if there is a shallow ledge that someone can be floated off of and returned to at the end.

Beginning at the Wall

Tell your partner to stand, back to the wall. Say, "Find the most comfortable position you can, leaning with your back flat against the wall. Spread your legs to give yourself a wide base. In a moment I'm going to float you out into the pool where you can let your back completely go. Before we start, focus on the straightness in your back. Feel how good it feels leaning against the wall. When the Watsu is near completion you will again feel the wall at your back. When you do, focus again on this feeling of straightness and whatever feeling of rising you feel up your back. When we have finished, stay as long as you want and feel free to let your body move whatever way it wants." Stand to the right. Place the right arm behind your back and the crook of your left elbow behind the neck. Your left knee is just under the right hip. Place your right hand on the heart chakra. Stay still a few breaths feeling your connection to the heart center. Lift your left knee under the hip to start floating partner away from the wall, your right forearm under the tailbone lifting toward the surface.

If you are in a pool that does not have a wall suitable to lean back against, start with the person standing out in the middle. Stand to the right, the right arm behind your back and under your left arm. Hold the heart center (the chest) between your hands. Coordinate breathing. Place your right arm under the sacrum and slowly lift up toward the surface, the head dropping back into the crook of your left elbow. Float partner close to your heart.

Basic Moves

a. Water Breath Dance

The right arm is under your left arm and behind your back. The occiput is comfortably settled into the crook of your left elbow. Your right forearm is under the tailbone (not under the lower back which could hyperextend it). Your hands are limp, palms and fingers downwards. The side of the chest is against your heart center. Stay low in the water, your legs spread as wide as is comfortable. You begin from the right so that your stronger right arm will have the greater burden if there is a tendancy to sink. If you are left handed, you can begin from the left. Don't try to hold someone out of the water, except for the nose, particularly if the air outside is cold. Hold still a moment. Feel how the water holds both of you. You are holding with your heart center. The water is holding you both as one. As you breathe out, slowly sink into the emptiness at the bottom of the breath. As you breathe in feel how it is the water breathing you both back up. Staying low in the water, continue this with each breath (your own), sinking and rising to whatever direction the Water Breath Dance takes you. Notice how letting your body go and surrendering this way is rocking the one in your arms. The freer the other's body becomes, the more your own body lets go. If partner is heavy, each time you breathe in let the water lift your right side, the side that brings partner closer to the surface. Notice what is, or is not, letting go. If the legs are stiffened, slip your right arm under the knees and lift gently to encourage them to bend. Then return to under the sacrum. If the weight is too much, move from this first position (Heart Float) before your right arm begins to tire, into the second (Open Arms), where it is easier to balance the weight.

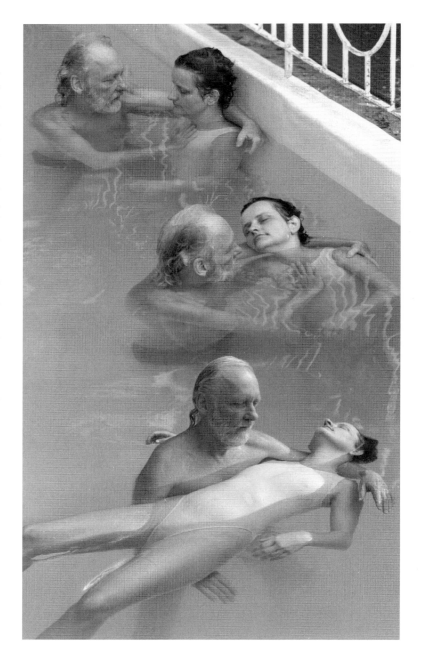

b. Open Arms

While rocking forward, the crook of your left elbow against the occiput, slip your right forearm under the knees. Balance partner between your arms, keeping them as open as is comfortable. Continue to sink and rise to whatever direction the water takes you. Notice how much lighter partner is in this second position, the weight evenly balanced between your arms. Let your body go more and more with each out breath.

c. Accordion

Each time you breathe out, let the middle of the body sink deeper. Notice if the knees gradually come closer to the chest on each outbreath without effort. If tightness or holding in the knees and/or hips restricts the folding inwards, gently bounce the knees up. Try maneuvering the torso into a more vertical alignment with each outbreath, encouraging the hips to fold by shifting the weight forward. If there is still holding, try rotating the near leg for a moment (bouncing and moving it if it's still tight) before returning to the accordion. As the knees come closer to the chest, notice the outbreath. Each time your arms come closer, stay longer at the bottom of the breath. Open your arms wider each time you both breathe in, feeling your own chest open. Avoid any extraneous movement that would distract from totally emptying into the bottom of the breath or fully opening.

d. Rotating Accordion

Continue opening and closing the 'accordion'. After each opening of your arms, lean forward, sweeping your right arm out over your partner's left side as you breathe out. After each closing, rock back and open your arms as you breathe in. This slowly rotates the two legs still in the crook of your right arm, releasing tension in the hips and lower back.

e. Near Leg Rotation

As you start to rock back to open your arms, let the far leg slip off your arm. Without breaking rhythm, lean forward to rotate the near leg up towards the left shoulder as you breathe out. Each time you rock back let yourself go even more, sinking back into the water. Co-ordinate your movement with your breathing, either bringing the leg up towards the opposite shoulder with each outbreath, or, if a slower rhythm seems more appropriate, breathing out when the leg is up and again when you are leaning back with it. Continue rotating the leg this way in the crook of your right elbow. Turn clockwise, the direction in which the water's resistance helps stretch the far leg.

When first learning these moves go on to the Completion described at the end of this chapter. Master each section and go to the Completion before returning to the pool to learn to combine it with the subsequent section.

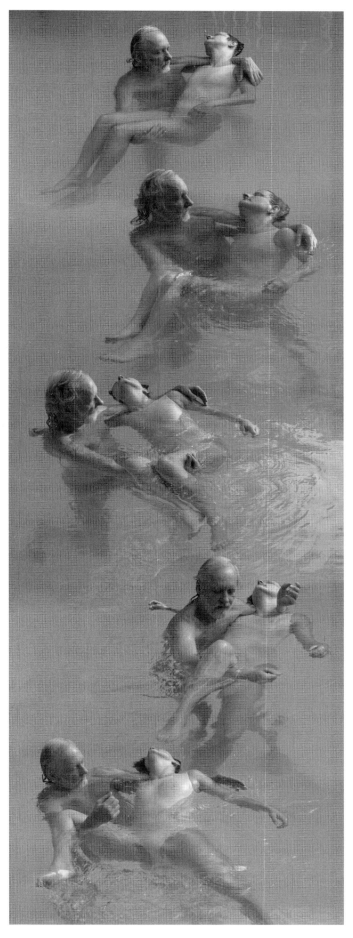

Section I The Head Cradle

In all three sections, the Basic Moves are followed by a cradle, which is followed by simpler positions. In first learning each section it is best to practice moving someone into and out of the simpler positions before learning the cradle that opens the section. Besides making it easier to learn the sections, this gives you a chance to practice in isolation those parts of each section which can be done by themselves when you get someone whose legs are not flexible enough to move into a cradle. Before learning the capture (a.) go into the pool and practice finding the 'float point', that point under the upper back where someone can be floated and balanced on one hand (the support of your forearm under the lower back can be added with those who sink). To find and use this center of buoyancy, begin by floating someone in the first position. Place your right hand, palm up, under the float point. Remove your left arm from under the neck and, with your left hand, slip the right arm out from behind your back. Once the arm is free between you, hold the head in your left hand and practice that part of the flow described below in f-h. Work from the first position into the Free Float, into the Under Head position, and back to the first position, over and over, until it flows smoothly. Once you master these transitions and positions, learn the Head Cradle from the beginning.

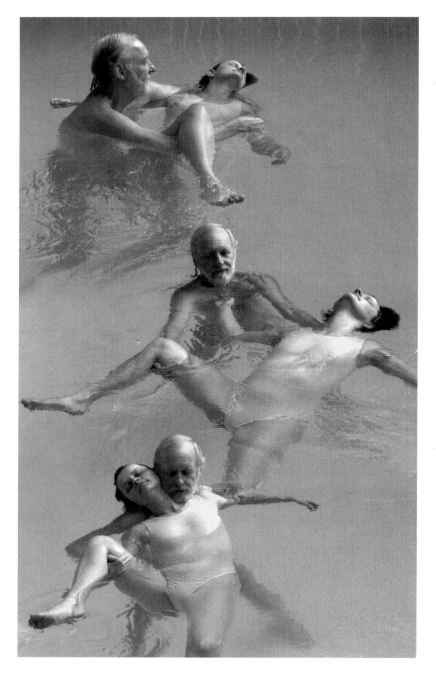

a. Capture

Open at the wall and do the Basic Moves. When the near leg is at the widest part of its rotation, keeping your left arm out straight, let the neck slip out your forearm and hold the head in your left hand. Hold the back of the right knee with the heel of your right hand between the two large tendons. Push the knee towards the chest turning partner onto the right side until the right arm slips free from behind your back. (If it doesn't come out by itself, straighten the right leg and float partner with your right hand under the float point in the upper back. Let go of the head and, with your left hand, pull the arm out from behind your back.) When the right arm hangs free in front of you under your right arm, the head in your left hand, stay low in the water and slip your right shoulder under the head, the back of the neck snug against your neck and shoulder. The head is on the same side of your head as your arm that is still holding the knee, the heel of your right hand still between its tendons, your fingers relaxed. (Hooking the heel of your hand under the knee, instead of grasping it with your fingers, helps keep your arm from tiring.) The right arm is still under yours. Do the above as one uninterrupted flow that leads into the following moves.

b. Arm-Leg Rock

As soon as you cradle the head, reach over the upper left arm, and, gripping it with your left hand, pull it back to your left side. Notice how this establishes the neck firmly against yours. Still holding the left arm, pull the right knee out to the right side. Pulling both arm and knee, rock turning from side to side. Co-ordinate your breathing to your turning, breathing in each time you pull the arm.

20

c. Twist

Slowly start moving the right knee towards the left side. Reaching under the left arm, replace your right hand under the knee with your left. Reaching over the shoulder, hold down the upper right corner of the chest with your right hand, while your left continues pulling the knee across. Gradually and gently twist stretch the spine, increasing the stretch slightly with each outbreath.

d. Knee Head

Let go of the right shoulder. Hold the head with your right hand. Your left hand is still under the right knee. Plant your left foot out in front of you and your right behind. Rock slowly from foot to foot to swing partner out and back.

e. Second Side

Let go of the right knee. Slip the heel of your left hand under the left knee and, keeping the left arm under your left arm, slip your left shoulder under the head. Work a mirror image of the above moves (b - d.), doing the Arm Leg Rock, Twist and Knee Head from the left side. After swinging your partner out and back, let go of the left knee and hold under the sacrum with your right hand.

f. Stillness

Hold the head in your left hand and the sacrum in your right, the right arm floating between you. This is the Free Float position. Both arms and legs float free. It is the best position in which to give someone a moment of absolute stillness. Let partner float perfectly still in front of you. Feel the stillness in your own body. If partner is heavy in your arms, try bracing your right elbow against your right hip. If that doesn't alleviate the problem, or if the water temperature is less than ideal, go right into the next move. Never stay in any position in which either of you might be uncomfortable.

g. Free Movement

Beginning slowly, rising and sinking with your breath, move partner freer and freer, getting your own body freer. Notice how freely the arms and whole body move in Free Float.

h. Hip Rock

Keep the arms in front of you. Slip your left shoulder under the back of the neck. Stay low in the water to give as much support to the neck as possible. Hold the hips with both hands and move freely from side to side with the breath. Don't let the lower back arch and hyperextend. After exploring movement in this position (Under Head), keep your right hand under the right hip while your left hand reaches down and slips the right arm behind your back to return to the first position.

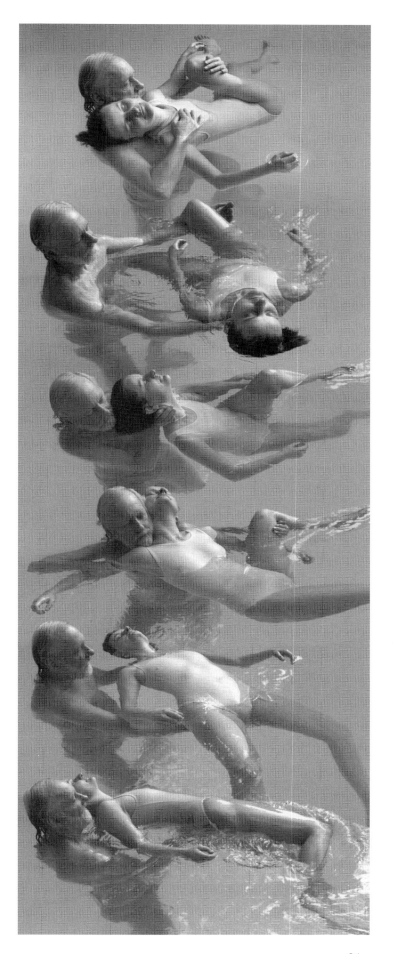

Section II Under The Far Leg, Shoulder and Hip

In learning the Basic Moves you learned two positions: Heart Float and Open Arms. In the First Section you learned two more: Free Float and Under Head. In this section you learn the last two of the six simple positions used in the flow: Under Shoulder and Under Hip. Practice these before tackling the Far Leg Cradle. What is 'under' in the last three of the six is your own shoulder, whichever is closest to your partner. To practice this section's simple positions first, begin with the Heart Float, and, using the float point, slip the arm that was under the neck under the near shoulder and do the moves described below in d - f, changing all lefts to rights and rights to lefts if you are starting from the right. Repeat this thoroughly on both sides before going on to learn the cradle that opens this section. Unlike the first section, in which you did the cradle on both sides, and then the simple positions on just one side, in this section, all moves are done first on one side, and then on the other.

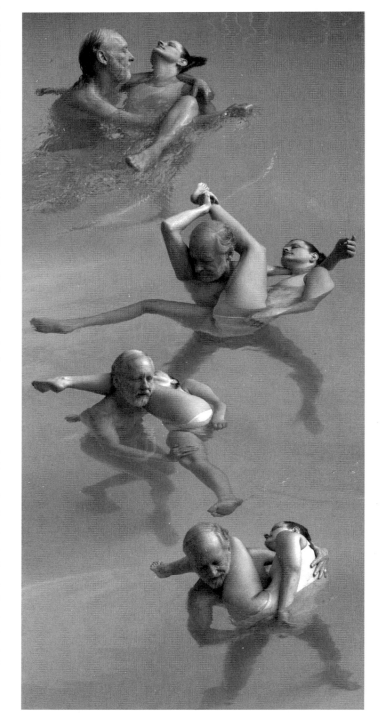

a. ⊗ Far Leg Over

Repeat the Basic Moves. Rotate the near leg out to its widest. Slip your right arm out from under it. Without breaking the rhythm of the rotation, lean forward and scoop up the far leg with the crook of your elbow under the knee. Rotate it in the same counter-clockwise direction as you did the near leg, bringing it up as close as possible to the far shoulder. Let the body move freely. When your arms are at their most open during the last rotation, reach out with your right hand and hold the right leg just above the ankle. Lift it up higher than your head, creating a space, a window between the back of the leg and your arm. Slowly pass your head through this space. Lower the leg, wrapping it around the back of your neck. Face away from the head to keep the leg from pressing against your throat. While your left hand keeps the head high enough to prevent the nose from going under, keep your shoulder low enough to minimize the weight on it.

b. Leg Push

Hold the upper back behind the heart center with your left hand, your left arm still under the head. With your right hand just above the knee, push the right leg out. As you push slowly turn clockwise so that the resistance of the water aids in stretching that leg.

c. Sacrum Pull

Bend the knee. Push the right leg down in front of you, across your abdomen, and around your waist. The back of the right knee should be snug against your side. While doing this, move your body in whatever way makes it easier for the leg to pass around you. Partner is still lying on the side. With your left hand pull the upper back, pressing the chest as close to the knees as possible. Hook the fingers of your right hand into the top edge of the sacrum and pull down to stretch open the lumbar spine. With your right hand push against the left hip. With your left hand lay partner back into the water without letting the head hang too far back in the process. Hold the float point under the upper back with your right hand. Slip your left shoulder out from under the left leg by lowering yourself in the water.

⊗ indicates difficult move that may need to be left out.

22

d. Under Shoulder

Staying low in the water, move under the shoulder with your right shoulder and, reaching up around the other side of the neck, place your right hand on the heart center. Your shoulder under partner's and your hand on the chest is what characterizes the Under Shoulder position. Keep your right elbow raised under the head, and the rest of your body as low in the water as possible, to keep the neck from stretching back too long.

e. Lengthening Spine

Support under the sacrum with your left hand. As soon as you hear or feel partner breathe out, let the lower body sink a little. As you both breathe in, slowly lift up and away from you by pushing your left hand against the top of the sacrum. Continue sinking and lifting with each breath. Your right hand very lightly presses down on the chest each time partner sinks, and keeps contact with the chest to provide traction to lengthen the spine each time you push against the sacrum.

f. Spine Pull

Holding the occiput in your right hand, straighten your right arm as you move down to the side, your left shoulder just under the left hip. This is what defines this as the Under Hip position. Hook the fingers of your left hand into the top of the sacrum. Pull to straighten and stretch the whole spine.

g. Undulating Spine

Stay low in the water close to, or just under, the left hip. With your left hand, palm up, under the sacrum, bounce on your feet to initiate wave movements up the spine, all the way up the neck which lies loosely in your right hand (your right arm still out straight under the shoulder). Hold under the float point with your left hand. Reach over the left arm and, holding the occiput in the crook of your right elbow, move into the first position on the second side.

h. Second Side

Do the Basic Moves on the second side. Rotate the far leg and do a mirror image of the above moves (a. - g.). When you return at the end to the first position on the first side, do the Basic Moves again.

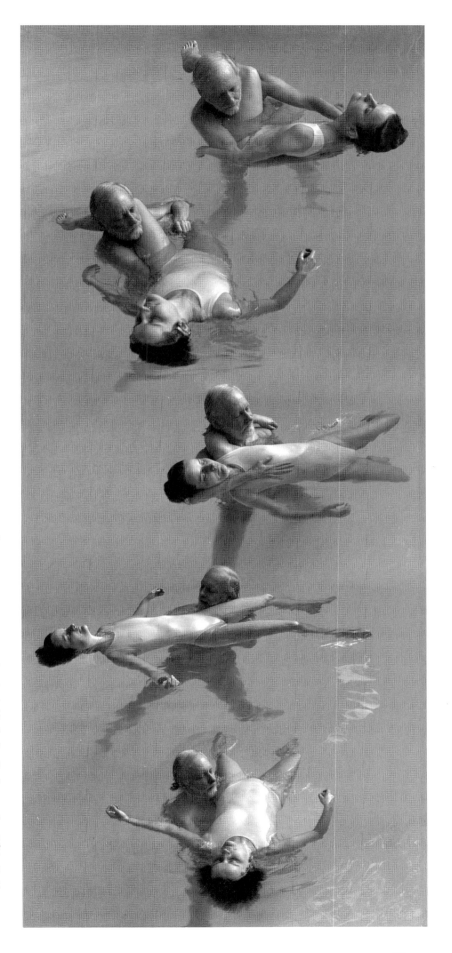

Section III The Near Leg Cradle

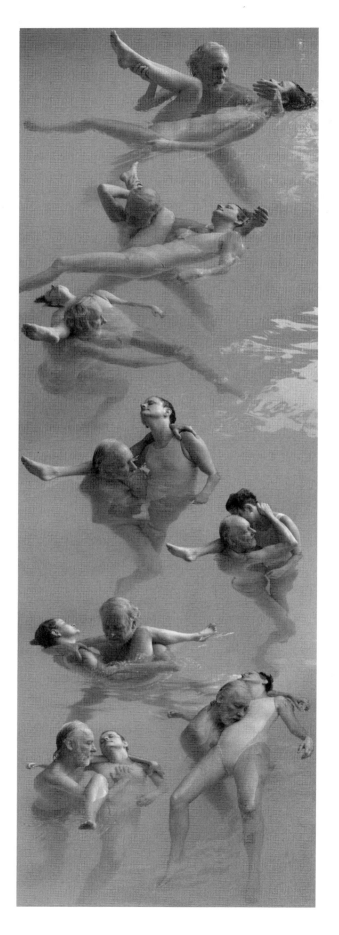

a. ⊗ Near Leg Over

Repeat Basic Moves. While rotating the near leg to its widest, take hold of it just above the ankle with your right hand. Stay low in the water. Wrap the near leg around your neck just as you did the far leg in the last section. Hold the occiput in your left hand.

b. Down Quads

Start at the top of the far leg. Grip the quadriceps muscles down the front between fingertips and heel of your right hand. Roll the leg. Slowly work down to over the knee (dont pull the kneecap).

c. ⊗ Leg Down

Push the far leg away from you with your right hand while very slowly turning clockwise (the direction in which the resistance of the water stretches the leg). Push the left leg down with your right hand while your left hand supports the back, swinging the torso up to a vertical position. (If the pool is so shallow that the left foot would hit the bottom, bend the leg at the knee before pushing it down.) Catch the knee against the inside of your right leg just above your knee, keeping it from slipping between your legs. Rest the forehead against the other knee that is still over your left shoulder. Hold the back with your right hand. Replace it with your left hand and, reaching over the left arm, hold the neck with your right hand. Lean into the lowered knee with your right leg while pulling the upper back towards you to stretch the whole body. Squeeze and work the neck with your right hand. Doing this with your right hand instead of your left, lessens the chance of the movement in your left shoulder irritating the tendons in the back of the knee. It also positions your right arm to receive the neck when you lower your partner.

d. Leg Pass

Step your left leg behind your right leg (which still has the left leg caught against it). Let the left leg rise towards the surface to your left. Lower the neck into the crook of your right elbow.

e. Arm

The right knee is still on your left shoulder. If the tendons in the back of it feel caught, shift your left shoulder slightly to slip them free. The right arm is in front of you. Squeeze it with both hands, pulling in opposite directions. Reach around and tug the left thigh with your left arm causing the right leg to slip off your shoulder. You are in the first position on the second side.

f. Second side

Repeating the Basic Moves again on the second side is optional. After tugging the left leg you can reach under and rotate it. Do a mirror image of all the above moves (a. - e.).

g. Heart Home

Back in position 1 on the first side, rock gently. Rest the side of your head on the heart center (facing away) and continue rocking with the breath. Lift your head up. Reach all the way under the near leg with your right arm and place your right hand on the chest where your head was without breaking the rhythm of the rocking. Continue to rock, your hand on the heart center.

Completion

In the following closure, you lean your partner back against the wall. If there is no suitable wall, you can finish on steps, or on a ledge, or on the shore. If none of these exist, you can stand someone in the middle of the pool, supporting with your hands on each side of the chest, holding the heart center until your partner is ready to stand alone. It is important to program people beforehand so that when the wall is behind, or the steps or ledge underneath, they know the Watsu has come to the finish. A clear separation at this point is equally important, as is your staying nearby to be there when the eyes open.

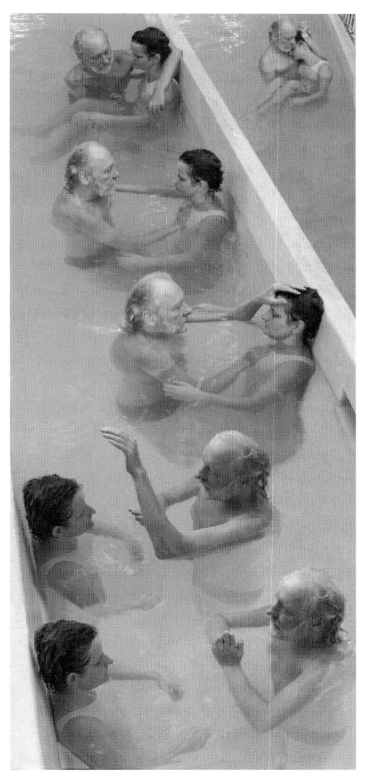

a. Wall Return

When you are ready to finish, slip your right forearm under both knees and bring them as close to the chest as possible. Stand high in the water, the head on the left corner of your chest, and rock slowly. Gradually approach the wall. As the back (still vertical) comes up flat against the wall, set partner on your left knee, which is out along the wall. Let the far leg slip off your right arm. Push it out away and pull the near leg toward you to create as wide a base as there was when you began from the wall. Hold neck and occiput with your left hand. Pull the spine up vertical if it is leaning to one side. Place your right hand on the heart center and, keeping both hands where they are, move out in front. Lean your knees against the knees. If comfortable, your two feet can be lightly over the toes or against the outsides of the feet. Stay holding this way, letting your own body settle comfortably in the water.

b. Lift Off

Let go of the neck a moment to see if the head stays up by itself. If it flops to one side (or if the pool is too deep), you can move to the steps or elsewhere to finish. If the neck is capable of supporting the head, gradually slip your left hand out from behind the neck. With your right hand still on the heart center, place your left hand lightly on the head, the heel over the third eye and the fingertips just touching the crown chakra. Keeping both hands in place, focus on the feeling of rising up your own back. When you feel it strongest, gradually lift both hands up. Slip them back into the water and with your fingertips lift up under the centers of the palms, lifting until your partner's hands almost break the surface. Draw your own hands out from under and press them together in front of your heart center, at the same time as you rock back on your heels withdrawing contact from the knees and feet.

c. Honoring the Space

Stay low in the water, your hands still pressed together in front of your heart center. Focus on how you can still feel the connection even though you are no longer touching. Feel how you are connected and separate. Honor the space between you. It is Heart space. Do not rush up to touch or hug. If the eyes are still closed, stay. Be there as they open.

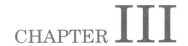

EXPLORATIONS

The following explorations of Watsu in writing occurred at various times during the long development of Watsu. In the one that follows you will find the first descriptions of those aspects of Watsu that will later become the basis of Rebonding Therapy.

Nurturing, Bonding, Intimacy and the Oneness Felt During a Watsu

The oneness felt during a Watsu creates a bonding reminiscent of both that between a mother and child, and the bonding between lovers. It creates a space safe enough to experience aspects that had been lacking in earlier bondings, as well as aspects that have been suppressed since painful separations. For many it is the discovery of a level of nurturing they have missed since childhood. It is the discovery of just how much intimacy we can enjoy without any sexual intention underlying it. Discoveries such as these have far reaching effects in a person's life and the quality of 'bonding' they will look for with others. It is imperative that the giver maintain a space within which the receiver can make these discoveries as safe as possible.

Non regression
For many people the fact they have not been held by anyone in their adult life the way they were held as a child has left a deep craving. Many deny a need exists. In Watsu, as that need is fulfilled, it comes into awareness and can be accepted. The strength and healing the child drew from that source are again available in his or her life. This should not be confused with 'regression.' It is the absence of regression, it is the not having to become a baby to find that source, it is the being able to find that nurturance in the here and now, which gives the experience such power.

Continuity
The same thing is true of the womb-like experiences many recipients mention. By being moved so freely through the water, by being repeatedly stretched and returned to a fetal position, the adult has the opportunity to heal in himself whatever pain or loss he may still carry from that time. If there is any sense of the restrictions his body grew into within the womb, he may now experience how free his body can be in water. If he has repressed any pain of separation, he can now feel the continuity, the oneness between that time and the present. It is not regression but creation, the power to create in one's own life a wholeness between the past and the present.

Intimacy
Watsu can also help heal wounds to our ability to accept intimacy, whether they were caused through a deprivation of physical contact, or through instances of childhood or later abuse. It can also help people reach a healthier understanding of their own sexuality.

Sexual feelings
Many problems people have around intimacy are related to their inability (or the people they choose as partners' inability) to distinguish between sexual feeling and sexual intention. Men, in particular, often have this difficulty. They have been trained that a sexual feeling is something to be acted on or repressed. The pressure to act causes them to fantasize a receptivity beyond what might be there. It prevents them from 'being' with another, fully sensitive and attentive to where the other is. In their focus on performance the other becomes

an object. The only other way they know how to handle a sexual feeling is to repress it. But repression divides the self, which also makes it difficult to completely 'be' with another.

The pleasure the whole body feels

There are ways of dealing with sexual feeling other than action or repression. This becomes clear during a Watsu where there is no place for sexual intention. In work this close, sexual feelings can come up, but, because there is no way to act on them, they can be enjoyed as pleasurable feelings in themselves, as part of the pleasure the whole body feels being moved continuously through the water. Uncompartamentalized, ungenitalized these feelings can contribute to the release and movement of energy throughout the body, particularly the movement of energy up the spine.

Becoming free of intention

Sexual intention propelled me into bodywork the day I walked up to a woman sitting beside a hot spring pool and asked her if she would like a massage (something I had never received in my life let alone given). But the more I worked with bodywork, and particularly with Watsu, the more I felt such connection and joy and fulfillment in the work itself that the imposition of any goal or sexual intention would be out of place. It would be a violation of the trust I felt the person placing in my arms. At the same time I began to feel powerful vibrations of energy rise up my own back, which at the end of a Watsu, would often combine with that of the person I had been working with and rise up over our heads. It was such a bright powerful experience that I began to look for, to anticipate it at the end of each Watsu. But that was substituting another goal, another intention, in place of just 'being' with the person. As I began to let go of that intention, I found that many similar and equally powerful events can occur anyplace during a session when there is no trying to make them happen. It is in this surrender to the moment that we free our bodies, and the more surrendered we become, the more surrendered and freer those we work with become.

The oneness

Many of those who receive a Watsu speak of feeling their bodies so completely supported and freed that they feel they are flying or sailing through space. Some speak of experiencing cosmic joy or unconditional love, other words for the oneness. My own strongest experience of this occurred this year in a class in Germany where, rather than feeling the rising up my back rise up to join the other's, there was only the one rising up the both of us. The whole pool, and all those around us, were bathed in its light.

Whatever the experience, because it is arrived at through the body's being freed (and not through its being denied), it is an experience that is incorporated in the here and now of the person's life.

Other intentional modes

There are other intentional modes besides the sexual that should be avoided during a Watsu. Some people may be tempted to play the parent too heavily, not allowing the receiver the freedom to move in and out of whatever state he needs to. Some may distance themselves by holding too close to a doctor/patient model. All such intentions and needs to control fall away as you feel your oneness with the person.

A celebration unfolding

So many people express either verbally, or in their face and body, how much they feel a 'oneness' in (and after) a Watsu that I am convinced that state of 'being at oneness' is crucial to our ability to free our bodies. It provides a context within which our individual limitations are no longer overwhelming. It gives us a new, more accepting perspective on our own and other's lives. In giving the Watsu, the more we feel at one with the other, the freer are our own bodies, and the more individual and unique each session becomes. The more we become one the freer we are to discover our uniqueness. It is as if our uniqueness can only truly unfold in our 'oneness'. And Watsu, at its most creative, becomes a spontaneous celebration of that unfolding.

Water is different to each

The water in which we do our Watsu, is itself a symbol of oneness, but when we look a little more closely at water, we see how unique the associations are each person has around it. Water is not the same thing to someone living in a desert as it is to someone who lives by the sea or in a rain forest or in a place threatened by devastating floods.

Different wombs

All of us began our existence in water. Water is the ideal medium for the developing fetus to explore the movement potential in its newly unfolding limbs. Its 'exercise program' begins as early as the eighth week. But being connected as we were to our mothers' emotional states, to her unique rhythms of adrenalin, endomorphine and other hormones and chemicals periodically flooding our common systems, our experiences of womb life are as different as are our mothers.

Water's roles in our lives

All of us experienced leaving that watery place, in one way or another. And water has since played so many roles in our lives: what we played and were bathed in, what our wounds were washed in, what many of us were baptized in, what we were warned not to go into by ourselves (especially after eating), what we almost drowned in, what we finally conquered and learned to float and swim in and under and on waves on top of.

Changing water

To the degree that what water means to us is the sum of all our individual experiences of it, this completely new experience, Watsu, changes what water is. To the degree that our past continues to live in us, this changed meaning reverberates back into and enriches all our memories in which water played a part.

In the same sense Watsu, and the oneness we feel in it, can change in us what it means to be with another; can enrich our understanding of all our relationships.

These changes are gained experientially and not 'intentionally'.

If we *intend* to change, if we set up a program for ourselves; if we tell ourselves that from this point on we are going to feel unconditional love or oneness with everyone, and then, as inevitably will occur, we feel some judgment or negative feeling toward others, we must suppress that feeling denying a part of ourselves, or feel guilty and inadequate.

Unconditional Love

With Watsu we feel connections with people that we might never have imagined feeling any connection. No matter what attitude you might have had toward someone, when you feel yourself letting go in their arms, or when, giving a Watsu, you feel someone surrendering, placing such trust in your arms, everything changes.

The more people we feel this unexpected connection with, the more we can free ourselves from the judgments and negative feelings that will still occasionally come up; the more accepting we can be of ourselves knowing how such attitudes dissolve in our 'oneness' in the water.

The Poetics of Watsu

Yesterday Bill Thomson, while interviewing me for an article on Watsu to appear in "East West Journal," pointed out that the group of San Francisco poets I was a member of in the late fifties and sixties were forerunners of today's consciousness raising movements. Exploring correspondences between then and now sheds some light on the origins and nature of Watsu.

The young poet

I can't imagine anyplace more exciting than San Francisco of the late fifties for a young poet. Besides the almost nightly getting together in the Place in North Beach, and the morning-afters on the lawn at Aquatic Park, there were the regular Sunday meetings where we would read each other our latest poems. I was addicted to writing, and to the state I would get into when a poem would come through on its own; a state I would characterize as one of absolute clarity; of writing with light. Nothing could compare to it. I shunned religion and family and the army and psychoanalysis and anything else I feared might undermine my being a poet (including drugs).

Isolation

But over the years as the North Beach 'scene' disintegrated in a haze of alcohol, I spent more and more time abroad (two years in Europe, one in Canada and three in Mexico). I no longer had the audience that the Sunday meetings and the White Rabbit and Open Space's publishing of my books provided. I became more and more isolated, an isolation all the more complete because the way I saw myself as a 'poet' set me above the lot of ordinary mortals. I wrote less and less.

When I discovered bodywork I found a way out of that isolation. I found in Watsu, a way to enter with others states similar to what I feel when the poem is coming through most clearly.

Correspondences

I see many correspondences between the poetics that evolved in the late fifties and what happens in Watsu. As poets, freeing the language from its habitual restrictions and limitations was uppermost, just as in Watsu freeing the body is. Both are based on the breath and free rhythms. Both seek places that open us up to possibilities beyond what we can anticipate. Influenced by Zen, both are practices that focus on the here and now, and get us in touch with the unknown. By advocating the kind of freedom they do, both find themselves in opposition to more traditional academic forms; and discover form by breaking through form.

A poem in motion

From the beginning I conceptualized Watsu as a sort of poem in motion. I can see my earlier habits of working over and revising poems reappear in the way I work out Watsu sequences for my students. I feel, when Watsu is freest, a creativity at play. This is extremely important in Watsu. There is a need, a drive for creativity in each of us. The more the giver works out of their creativity, the more the receiver feels areas open up that might not have been otherwise accessed. When we move beyond our conscious mind and let go of its need to control, something takes over that knows on a much deeper level just what is needed in the other (who is no longer so much an 'other').

Freeing body, heart and mind

Seeing the origins and effects of Watsu partially embedded in this drive for creativity complements two other aspects of its origin I have already written about: the physical and the emotional (the need for connection with others). Those first two are body and heart, and this third (and the clarity that characterizes it) is mind. Watsu's movement, its dance, frees the body. The closeness and nurturing of Watsu free, and open the heart. And its inventive play and spontaneity free the mind.

In the Boundlessness of Water

They yielding water

Water's strength is in its power to yield, to flow into whatever form would pretend to contain it, to move over and make room for whatever enters it. What better medium could we find in which to learn whatever we need to learn about yielding? In Taoist philosophy this yielding of water is the 'role model' for all our activities, or rather 'non activities' in the world.

Chaos

The study of the movement of water is the basis of a new science, the science of chaos, which has uncovered a kind of recurrent pattern that seems common to all chaotic events. The freer we get in water, moving with someone, never repeating the exact same movement twice, the more it feels we are moving to a similar kind of 'chaotic' pattern. That pattern might itself facilitate some of the remarkable changes of consciousness experienced during a Watsu. It echoes the chaos that, in so many mythologies, underlies creation and is described as 'the face of the deep', the sea.

Boundaries

Another way water affects our consciousness is what it does to our sense of boundary. This varies dramatically with changes in the temperature of the water. In cold water when the pores of our skin close and the capillaries contract there is a heightened sense of our boundary, and the cold it is trying to keep out from the warmth within. In contrast, when the water is the same temperature as our skin (as it is ideally in Watsu), our pores open and our capillaries dilate, as our body feels more and more boundless.

The five sheaths

I am reminded of the five sheaths that surround the atman, the self, in India. Underlying the food sheath, that which we feed and is itself food (for worms and vultures . . . and fire), is the sheath of prana, the warmth, the fire within. Underlying this is the mental sheath, that which sorrows for the body's pain and rejoices in its pleasure. Under this is the wisdom sheath, the innate wisdom of the body. And under this, the sheath of bliss, the rapture that is the foundation of our lives.

Rapture

The boundlessness felt in warm water is the sheath of prana, the warmth within, becoming one with the warmth of the water. During a Watsu, when our mind's chatter becomes most stilled, the more spontaneous and intuitive our moves become, the more they are coming out of our bodies' innate wisdom, and the deeper we move into rapture.

It is said that once an opening is made to the rapture, once we know how to access it, we will be able to see it underlying even the greatest of our sorrows. I can imagine no better goal for Watsu than to help people realize a level of consciousness from which they can face anything, a level as boundless as water.

Watsu and Continuum

*Breaking the
neural lock*
I have just come back from a weekend workshop with Emily Conrad Da'oud, the developer of Continuum. I was impressed with the parallels between what she is doing on land and what we are doing in water. In Continuum emphasis is placed on breaking the 'Neural Lock' that limits our movements to those habitually repeated over and over. Movements outside the habitual provide more neurological information and stimulate the organism. They counter the aging process that accelerates whenever our bodies become locked in habitual patterns. To break those patterns she had us explore both primitive movement and micro-movements. We carry in our bodies the whole history of evolution. When we go into our most primitive movements, the aquatic, we are on our most creative level.

*Movement as
prayer, as love*
She feels that when we learn and repeatedly practice a set form of movement as with most Yoga and Tai Chi, etc., we are practicing the conclusion of someone else's research, rather than discovering in ourselves those spontaneous movements that express where we are in our own bodies at this moment. Anything less separates us from ourselves. She sees movement that arises out of this deepest level as prayer, as love.

*Moving from a
shared space*
When the watsuer is most deeply connected to his partner, movement does arise out of this level, with a spontaneity and freedom that do not come from either body alone, but from a shared space. The more we watsu from this place, the more neurological information floods both our bodies, and the freer we are to move from within our own bodies when we separate.

I have found over the years that the stretches and meditations I have been doing with my classes have more and more come to incorporate and conclude with getting in touch with the spontaneous movement in the body. How important these Meditation Movements are to Rebonding Therapy has become clearer after studying with Emily. I recommend her courses to anyone interested in Watsu.

Sharks and Incest

Abuse
The warm pool in which Watsu was first developed at Harbin Hot springs draws people from all over the world. It also occasionally attracts a shark. A Watsu shark is someone, usually a male, who uses Watsu as a way to meet and seduce members of the opposite sex. It may be someone who has picked up a few moves by watching, or someone who has studied Watsu and somehow missed its basic principle of being, not doing. It used to be my assumption, that anybody learning and practicing Watsu would feel, as I do, such a connection that it would drown out any tendency to exploit the person in their arms. This is usually the case, but there have been exceptions. Over the years three or four men have been asked to leave Harbin and never come back. The shark net has been drawn tighter and tighter. It is rare that a shark of the first order turns up, someone who openly or surreptitiously violates the sanctity of someone's body while floating them.

*Sharks of the
second order*
Less rare are sharks of the second order, those who circle around and come back to their victim after having left them at the wall. These predators exploit the state Watsu leaves someone in. After receiving a Watsu, after having been held and nurtured in ways they haven't been since infancy, someone may be ready to follow the giver and acquiesce to whatever is asked to keep that connection and express their gratitude. But asking for anything after giving a Watsu puts a price on a gift and undermines all the benefits the person received from feeling someone just being with them. In Watsu people are open and vulnerable. They reach new levels of trust. They may overcome barriers set up by a history of abuse and incest, barriers that could come crashing back down around them, if the one stranger they could entrust their body to because the connection felt free of intention, comes back at them with intention. Even if someone acquiesces and seems to enjoy whatever sexual activity is

initiated, there is a good chance they will have a delayed reaction, the kind of pain, the shame that follows any other kind of incest. It is essential to hold the space around Watsu sacred.

New Dimensions

This is not to deny or downgrade sexuality. It, too, is sacred. There is nothing wrong with having sexual feelings while giving a Watsu, as long as there is no intention behind them, and the energy they generate moves up to the heart and higher without making any demands on the receiver. Giving Watsu is a wonderful way to train yourself to move that energy up. At the same time it trains you to hold the space of others in the highest regard. This training can improve your relations with others outside the pool and open up new dimensions to your sexual life. If ego or intention prevents you from being with others this way in Watsu, you miss an opportunity to enrich your life in a way that pursuing immediate gratification never can.

Be clear

Have no ulterior motive if you offer someone a Watsu. Have no intentions, no expectations. Watsu is an instrument of great power, loving power, which, if misused, cuts all the deeper. Be clear.

Under Water

Going under with Veechi

In the early years of Watsu, Veechi came from Montreal to study Watsu. In exchange she showed us Mouvance, the water work she had been developing. She massages people as they float with the help of devices under their head and around wrists and ankles. She also works with face masks which both wear. She holds the person, connecting her breathing to theirs, and goes under the water with them. As the person gets used to being taken under and relaxes, she watches for tension in their body and moves them in ways to release it. One move I particularly enjoy is one in which she holds a person by the ankles and moves their whole body in waves. My favorite of all her work is the way she has us partner up, each keeping responsibility for his or her own breathing, and take turns surrendering to each other. The spontaneity, the changes from a passive role: letting your body be moved freely, to an active role where you are moving the other, is quite joyful, is dolphin play.

Limitations under water

Floating devices, particularly under the neck, can be useful if you are working with a sinker much bigger than you, but otherwise I find they get in the way in Watsu. Though I enjoy the work under the water, particularly as partners switching roles, we have put off pursuing it here at Harbin because it is not as appropriate as Watsu in pools where a quiet meditative atmosphere is mandated. Also, underwater bodywork is not as accessible to the general public as Watsu. I can't imagine as many people being able to take each other under on their first day, and getting as much out of it, as they do in their first day's Water Breath Dance. Rather it is something for a specialist, requiring more training, sensitivity and practice, before you are able to put someone at ease for the greater surrender it requires. This was brought home to me on my last trip to Germany.

Being pushed under

When I arrived in Germany my students were talking about a new form of water work that combined Watsu and underwater work called Wassertanz (Water Dance). I wanted to experience this new work. In my second intensive, a student who said that she practiced it offered me a session. After floating me around the pool, she put a device on me that clamped my nose closed. She pushed me under, moved me around, and brought me up over and over. The rhythm at which she worked seemed to have nothing to do with my need to breathe and I felt moments of real panic, wondering when she was going to bring me up. I wondered if this panic was supposed to be part of the process. Another thing that made me wonder was the way her hand occasionally brushed across my genitals as she pushed me down, a kind of contact we never make in Watsu where it would be too big a distraction, but maybe here the distraction is not unwelcome, if it takes one's mind off being drowned. But one thing I couldn't imagine as part of the process was the pain, the way the clamp hurt, hurt so much that, finally, I had to take it off my nose. Afterwards I asked her where she had learned to do that. She said she hadn't actually studied Wassertanz herself but her boyfriend had, and he had showed her a few moves to which she added some of her own.

31

Wassertanz One evening during my next intensive, my students showed me a video made by Aman Schroter and Arjana, the Swiss couple who developed Wassertanz. With the underwater camera work, the supple movement of Arjana's dancer's body was quite beautiful. The session began with him standing in the middle of the pool, floating her, doing many of the moves of Watsu, but with his own body standing straight in the water while he worked. Then he held her and moved her around under the water, without going under the water with her the way Veechi does. He did the same wave motion Veechi does when she holds the ankles. I felt I was watching a combination of Watsu and Veechi's work in which the most essential element had been left out, that of freeing one's own body, of getting down into the water and being with the other.

Doing is required In my next intensive, a student who had studied with Aman gave me a Wassertanz. I still missed having someone going under with me the way Veechi does, but I felt he was more in synch with my breathing, though there were still a couple of times I was wondering when he was going to bring me up. And one time, while pushing me straight down, he lost his grip and my head hit the bottom. I could see it requires more doing, more muscular effort and size advantage, than Watsu. The wave and some of the other movements felt good, but I was continuously aware of not breathing and breathing. And the clamp was again putting my nose in a great deal of pain.

Returning underwater In my last intensive Aman and Arjana showed up to study with me. I asked Aman if he had ever studied Watsu or Veechi's work. He said he had studied Watsu through my first book and video, but that he had never encountered Veechi's work. I liked Aman and welcomed the opportunity to show him how Watsu has evolved to emphasize the freeing of one's own body and sinking into the breathing. When I mentioned that my experiences of Wassertanz were dominated by a constant awareness of whether I was breathing or not, he said people lose that awareness after a few sessions. He offered me a session, but there was no time before my return to America. This year Arjana came to Harbin to continue her studies of Watsu. She gave me a session which has renewed my appreciation of the potentials of underwater work. She sensitively took me past any hang-up with breathing and lung collapse to a point where I felt completely at home under the water, to where I became water. I felt it most strongly in my pelvis, which was freer to move than when someone is floating me on the surface.

Arjana's Water Dance Arjana introduces Water Dance to people after they've had at least three sessions of Watsu. This allows them to first experience how everything that comes up can be let go into the flow of a complete Watsu, and to build up the trust required for the greater surrender demanded by Water Dance. Her work is a valuable adjunct to Watsu. Arjana is developing a program of optional underwater work which will be integrated with our Watsu program in a manner which insures that the student first masters the art of being with someone on the surface, before attempting the more difficult art of being with them underwater.

Pools I Have Stepped Into

Adapting Teaching Watsu, stepping into pools all around the world, I've learned how much you have to adapt and make do with whatever is at hand, whether it's a swimming pool in Montparnasse with fifty watsuers or a hot tub on a boat in Amsterdam. Alongside depth and temperature, a third critical factor is ambience. This is effected by the amount of chlorine in the water, the people around, and the noise and flurry of jets, sprays, and man made currents. I remember one particularly active day at the big spa in Baden Baden where there didn't seem to be any part of the pool not hit by a jet or a spray and my class was stared at with murderous indignation by a family of immigrants from some culture where holding each other must not be ok. Nevertheless the class enjoyed itself that day, and maybe that family did too.

*Inside
another's head*

There is no saying what is going on inside someone else's head. One of my students had someone walk up to her while she was giving a Watsu and tell her to stop, that she would frighten children, who, if they saw someone lying so still in her arms, would think he was dead. Another student was told by the management at a spa that his watsuing of a man was disturbing the clientele (watsuing a woman would be ok.) Another time while a Watsu (in bathing suits) was being videotaped, someone went to the manager and complained about the pornographic film being shot in the pool. It is all in the eye of the beholder. There are people who are more threatened and confused by tenderness than by whatever sexual content they can project. We must not allow that to interfere with our ability to give others what we have to give. I've seen many people affected positively by just being around Watsu. Many have told me how calm it made them feel, how just watching put them into a meditative state. Many in the pool spontaneously start to float each other.

*Surrounding
our circle*

Each pool is different. At another spa in Germany we started as a small circle at the relatively quiet center of a big pool. As I demonstrated, a crowd of people began to gather around slowly closing in on us. The next thing I knew they were swinging their arms up over their heads all together, and then straight out to the sides. It was the six o'clock exercise class. We slipped outside.

No bottom

A more serious pool was one in Austria where I was the only one who could touch bottom. My organizers brought large plastic triangular blocks, but they floated up. They filled them with steel rods, but when someone stood on the blocks they slid around. Straddling two was dangerous. The water had so much chlorine in it everybody's skin was burning. And it was nowhere near warm enough. Finally by the third day it was almost tolerable. But when we came in the next day expecting to find it warm, it was cold. The owner, fearing for the cleanliness of his pool, had added fresh water (and more chlorine) the night before. I will never forget that pool.

*Drifting
together*

But there are many other pools we've been in that are truly unforgettable. I remember the snow covered Alps looming over the huge hot spring pool around the lake from Geneva, steam rising around us. I remember the 22 midwives watsuing each other in a line across the pool outside Venice. I remember the pool in the old people's home in Munich where our last class ended with everybody blissfully floating and drifting together into the corner under a window, the snow falling.

Stepping Out Of The Pool

*Watsu opens
the chest*

The other day in the warm pool someone told me what he found most remarkable in his first Watsu was the way it opened up his chest. He was a massage therapist and had been receiving bodywork for years. He had never had anything affect the intercostals (the muscles between the ribs) the way Watsu did. He pointed out that so much bodywork on land compresses the body whereas Watsu opens it. Besides those actual moves of Watsu that open the chest, and the weightlessness in water, I imagine this effect is enhanced by the way the breath fills the whole body during a Watsu, internally massaging it at the same time the warm water externally massages the body. This opens another line of exploration since the surface of our body, our skin, has in our development originated from the same level as our nerve tissue. It is our brain turned inside out, or rather our brain is our skin turned outside in. Both are being watsued through a sea of feelings and thoughts as broad and limitless as the sea someone steps into when they try to write about something as multidimensional and flowing as Watsu. These explorations could go on forever. Which makes this as good a point as any to step out of the pool and explore how the body can be freed on land. Land is a place where we can get more precise as to just how to feel and hold points and chakras, etc., knowledge that will serve us in good stead when we step back into the pool later in this book.

CHAPTER IV

WATSU ON LAND

When we leave the water, Watsu's nurturing power can be carried up on land. Its flow can enter all our bodywork. And what we learn on land can be carried back into the water.

Tantsu

As I developed Watsu, the more complete it became, the more I wanted to duplicate its power on land. I explored ways a giver could use his own body to cradle someone while stretching meridians, and holding chakras and points, ways the work could flow from cradle to cradle on land. The form that developed out of these explorations is called Tantsu (Tantric Shiatsu). Besides providing all the benefits that Shiatsu does, Tantsu takes both giver and receiver into states of meditation, energy and awareness that are as powerful as those experienced in the practices of Tantra.

Free Form

Both Watsu and Tantsu are rooted in our deepest impulse to free the body. In Watsu this impulse leads into what I call Free Flow. In Tantsu, as our bodies become freer, sometimes a gentle rocking, a slow wave like movement, carries us along as if the sea itself were under and around, as if we were the sea. One move flows into the next without intention in this form of bodywork, or state of being, that I call Free Form. Both it and Free Flow are free. They cannot be purchased. They are a gift. If we try to make them happen, they won't. The more you practice and know in your body all the forms of Watsu and Tantsu, the more you will be ready to let go of them whenever these moments of freedom appear. Knowing the forms; knowing in your body what you can do at any point; knowing that wherever the flow takes you there will always be something your body knows to do, frees you from looking for what to do next; frees you to let go into the unknown.

The ideal closeness

When I developed Tantsu, I taught it to students who had first learned Zen Shiatsu, who would consequently have a traditional form to use when the greater closeness of Tantsu was inappropriate. Just as the ideal pressure to apply to each point, and the ideal pull for each stretch, varies from individual to individual, so does the ideal closeness at which a practitioner should work. Knowing both Zen Shiatsu and Tantsu, and how to combine them, provides a range within which each session can be individualized.

Co-centering

To lighten the burden on the beginning student I developed a form that maintains a traditional distance while incorporating Tantsu's focus on chakras. Heart and body centers are connected, worked out from, and returned to over and over in a way that trains the beginner to connect breathing and to work from his own center. Because it centers both giver and receiver, it is called Co-Centering. Basic Co-Centering is simple enough to learn in a day, but powerful enough to practice repeatedly without exhausting its effectiveness. Like Watsu's Transition Flow, it becomes a framework when it is expanded. My book *Bodywork Tantra* presents this basic form, showing how it can be expanded to include the moves of Zen Shiatsu. It also presents basic and expanded forms of Tantsu.

Basic Tantsu

In this book, a single form, Basic Tantsu, integrates Co-Centering (in the face down position) and those moves of Tantsu that can be done with almost anybody. Like Watsu's Transition Flow it has a completeness, and a potential for connection that will never be exhausted, no matter how many times it is repeated. It, too, has been developed and fine tuned in countless classes here and in Europe and becomes a framework that can be expanded (with moves from *Bodywork Tantra*). Besides showing you how to cradle with your body on land, Basic Tantsu develops your ability to feel in your own center when you have connected with a point, and just how long it should be held, a skill that will be of value when you go back into the water to expand your Watsu.

Zen Shiatsu

Creative bodywork

The ultimate source of all the forms in this book is Zen Shiatsu. It was developed in Japan in this century by Shizuto Masunaga, the author of *Zen Shiatsu*. He integrates a variety of oriental techniques and healing modalities. Most traditional schools of Shiatsu emphasize thumb pressure on points. Masunaga has us use our whole body to work with the other's whole body. We use our forearms, elbows and knees, as well as our thumbs. Zen Shiatsu incorporates stretches, manipulations, and ampaku work on the hara. It emphasizes being with another rather than doing something to them. This presence is manifested in the connected breath and the use of the Mother Hand, the hand, or elbow or knee, etc., that stays in one place, providing constant support, while the other works, a presence that is essential to help balance the energies. Masunaga says more is happening under the hand that stays in one place than in the one that is working. Zen Shiatsu's eclecticism, its openness to a range of techniques and its emphasis on Zen presence and spontaneity, makes it the most creative of all oriental bodywork.

Developing unique styles

I went to Japan and studied with Masunaga the last year he taught. I had previously studied with his two students who first brought Zen Shiatsu to America, Reuho Yamada and Wataru Ohashi. I saw in the way each of these two had developed their own unique style, testimony to the creative power of Zen Shiatsu, and encouragement to plunge in when I began to transpose its principles and moves into water; and when I began to bring what I found in the water back up on land.

Tantsu

Bodywork Tantra

If Watsu were Zen Shiatsu in water, there would be no need for Tantsu. Watsu on land would be Zen Shiatsu. But holding someone in water puts us on a different level of intimacy than is present in Zen Shiatsu. It is a level on which we feel a greater opening and connection in all our chakras, a level on which we can come into a greater awareness of the energy that rises up our spine, and how it connects with another's. The power of such experiences prompted me to explore how Watsu and related bodywork are non-sexual forms of Tantra. In my book, *Bodywork Tantra*, I draw upon my own experiences of Tantra, and the correspondences between all its forms.

The first chakra

In water, with water's help, we truly hold the whole person. With water's help, there is contact with every chakra. In the expanded Watsu there are optional positions in which we cradle someone at our waist, or on our knee. These positions provide non-invasive support to the first chakra, which is in the perineum, while we work with the rest of the body, stretching and releasing points and meridians. The first chakra almost never receives this kind of non-sexual contact, this presence without intention. A great deal of tension is often locked there. It is the base of all our energy.

Out of the water

Tantsu brings this level of non-sexual intimacy and support up on land. In Tantsu, we use our whole body to hold and cradle someone throughout a session. These nurturing positions are sequenced in such a way that our support of the first chakra is gradually and non-threateningly introduced. The receiver remains clothed. Contact is limited to that part of our body supporting the other's as we focus on stretching and releasing meridians and major points. There is a Watsu-like flow throughout a session as we move someone from cradle to cradle without ever losing contact. The support is continuous and total. Tantsu is orchestrated so that at the finish whatever energy has been released during the session is focused up the spine. It ends with a separation in which both freedom and a sense of connection are as present as at the end of a Watsu.

BASIC TANTSU

The sequence

This sequence can be done with anyone who does not have a condition that precludes pressure or stretching. It opens with work on the back that is the same as in Co-centering. This Face Down position is followed by Tantsu cradles, a combination that gradually introduces the levels of intimacy, and allows you to perfect the use of your own body. Co-Centering trains you to lean in from your center. Tantsu develops your ability to hold with your center (When you hold with your center, the places you hold, no matter how far apart, become one). The work itself is meditation. The Movement Meditations at the end of this book help prepare you for this work. A shorter meditation which we use on the first day of our classes is included below. It helps you develop the ability to completely empty into the bottom of the breath, an emptying you can feel when you lean into someone or hold a point.

Learning as Process

Those first learning can profit by following an order we have developed as a process in our Watsu intensives. Before laying hands on anyone, practice the above meditation until you feel an emptying, a peace, that will carry over into your work. Learn first the Face Down sequence leaving out all the moves whose letters are surrounded by brackets [ ]. This way you first concentrate on connecting to another's breathing and leaning in from your center. Practice this abbreviated sequence, and the finish (Section VII), over and over until it feels completely natural, until you feel you are always working from the emptiness in your center. Then learn to add one by one the bracketed moves working with first, elbows, then, thumbs. By learning to work first with the heels of our hands and our elbows, which do not have the same habitual connection to the brain as our thumbs, it becomes easier to work from our center when we start using our thumbs. Next, learn the Head Cradle (Section IV), which is an ideal introduction to holding someone with your center. Then learn to incorporate the cradles from Section II to Section VI as they appear in this book. Next learn the Hara; and, finally, The Cradle of the Second Side which will introduce you to working with a greater freedom that can lead into Free Form.

Empty Center Meditation

Sit on the floor in whatever position helps keep your back straight, your hands in front of your hara, one hand cupped in the other, the tips of your thumbs touching. Focus on how your breath empties into your center as you breathe out, and rises up your back as you breathe in. That rising up your back is a wave spreading out to all parts of your body ... and all those parts let go and settle and empty into your center each time you breathe out. The whole area around the center, the navel the front, the sacrum the back, and the perineum the bottom, is a bowl at the base of the spine. Every time you breathe out everything empties into that bowl. At the very bottom of the breath, when everything has emptied into that bowl, the bowl itself empties. When everything has emptied into that bowl, the bowl itself empties into that point at the bottom, which is the first chakra, which is where our energy returns into the void, which is its most powerful state because it's pure potential. The more completely you empty into that point at the bottom of the breath, the more you can feel rising up your back as you breathe in. Feel that emptying and rising with each breath. Keep that emptying and rising and get up on all fours, hands and knees comfortably spread. Each time you breathe out feel the emptying in your center as you slowly rock forward. And each time you breathe in feel the rising up your back as you rock back, but not so far back that any effort is required to rock forward as you breathe out. Continue rocking with the breath this way, your arms straight, your back and neck relaxed. As you feel the emptying in your center feel how gradually your weight rocks into your hands on the floor. Sit back on your heels. Sit in the emptiness.

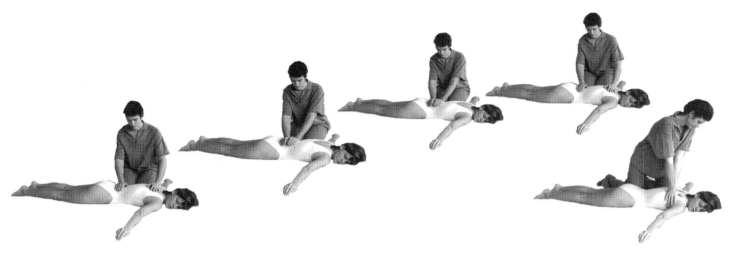

I Face Down

Make sure there are no conditions pressure or stretching might aggravate. Have your partner lie face down, arms comfortably out to the sides, head turned. If it makes the neck more comfortable, place a rolled towel under the upper chest. (If someone is not comfortable lying face down, do not use this position. Begin with the Leg Cradle and work on the back in the side position.) Tell partner to feel free to turn the head, and to let you know if anything is uncomfortable. Kneel to the left, facing, but not touching, the lower back. Sit on your heels (seiza). If your knees are uncomfortable, use a cushion between your legs to sit on. If your ankles are uncomfortable, place a rolled towel under them. Center. Look at the back. Observe the breathing.

a. Opening Rock

Simultaneously place your left hand over the spine between the shoulder blades (the back of the heart center) and your right hand over the lower back just above the sacrum (the body Center). Let your hands rest three breaths. Connect to the breathing. On an inbreath place your left hand alongside your right. As partner breathes out lean the heels of both hands into the muscle on the near side of the spine. Lean toward but don't touch the spine. With the next outbreath hook your fingers into the corresponding muscle on the other side and rock back. Sitting on your heels, arms and back straight, rock from your center and gradually build up speed. (Don't try to stay connected to the breathing.) Keep your hands in the bowed curve that best fits the back, that allows you to rock the heels of your hands into the muscle on this side, and hook your fingers into the muscle on the other side, without having to change the shape of your hands. Effortlessly, your fingertips lift slightly as you rock forward, and your heels lift as you rock back. When the rocking feels complete, when the spine feels the freest, hook your fingers in a fraction of an inch higher up the muscle each time you rock, causing your left hand to slowly walk up the back. When it has walked up a third of the way, jump it back and let it walk up a little farther. Let it walk up a third time, slowing down to rest between the shoulder blades, the rocking becoming slower and slower in your own center. As both hands rest on the heart and body centers, feel the stillness in your center. Feel the connection of the centers under your hands. Stay at least three breaths.

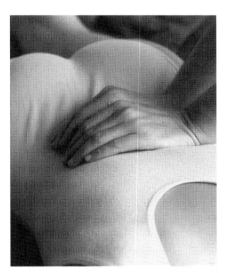

b. Both Hands

Get up on your knees, spread to give you a wide base, and face the opposite shoulder. Place the heels of both hands alongside the spine over the heart center, fingers pointed outward. Say "Take a deep breath and let it all the way out." As partner breathes out, breathe out, leaning in with both hands, slowly following to the bottom of the breath. Keep pressure vertical, perpendicular to the surface, intense, but not painful. Hold until partner is ready to breathe in. As you both breathe in, glide your hands a few inches down the back, and, when ready to breathe out, lean in again. Feel the emptying in your center. Repeat one more time at the bottom of the rib cage. Don't lean in with two hands where there are no ribs to support the spine.

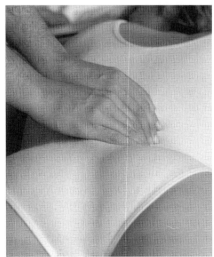

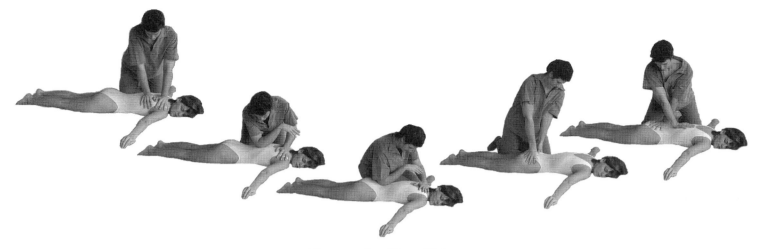

c. Down the Far Side

Facing the back, knees spread, place the heels of both hands to the other side of the spine, between it and the scapula. Your left hand, the mother hand, which should not be close to the neck, maintains a constant pressure midway between the zero and full pressure of the other hand. On the outbreath rock forward, leaning into your right hand. On the inbreath place the heel of your right hand further down and repeat. Lean altogether into three places along a line about an inch from the spine, evenly spaced between the heart center and the sacrum. If you are not going to use your elbow, lean into the same three places two more times.

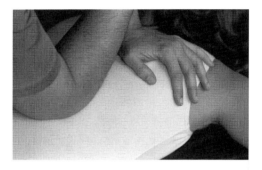

[d]. Elbows down Far Side

Before using your elbow for the first time, get to know it by placing it in your palm. Unlike your thumb, it can move freely around because of its loose skin. It finds its way into the points. An open elbow is less sharp. Keep your mother hand over the heart center. Lean an open elbow into points down the same line the heel of your hand has been leaning into (the Bladder meridian). As with the hand, feel the letting go in your center each time your elbow bottoms out in a point. Ease up if the person tenses. Get feedback. Keep it gentle. Adjust your own position as often as needed to stay comfortable. The last point is just before the sacrum.

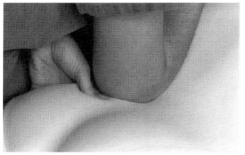

e. Down the Near Side

Moving far enough back to give yourself room to rock your weight forward, place both heels to the near side of the spine and lean into the three corresponding places, and in the same way, as down the far side.

[f.] Elbows down Near Side

If comfortable, sit on your knees alongside the back, and, with your mother hand on the heart center, ease into each point. Feel the letting go in your center which, rather than over the back, is now alongside.

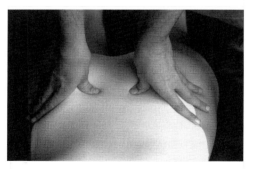

[g.] Thumbs down Sacrum

Your elbow in the last point before the sacrum, reach behind your elbow and place your left thumb in the highest indentation on the sacrum. Place your right thumb in the same point on the opposite side. Get up on your knees. Keeping arms straight, lean into points in the foramen down the sacrum. Finish leaning into points to each side of the tailbone.

h. Crossed Arm Stretch

Lay your left hand across the sacrum and, crossing over your left arm, place your right hand on the spine where it arcs the highest behind the heart. As you both breathe out, lean in with the heels of both hands, pushing apart, to gradually lengthen and stretch the spine. Hold until ready to breathe in.

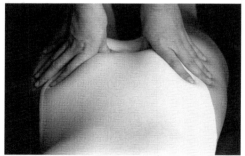

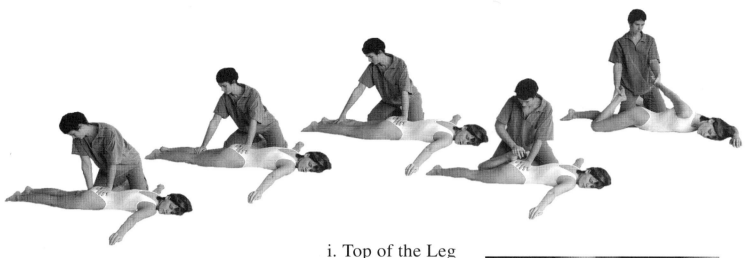

i. Top of the Leg

Without lifting your left hand off the sacrum, lean the heel of your right hand into the middle of the thigh at the top of the leg (the base of your thumb against the sitsbone). Hold three breaths (Bladder 50). Ride over the breath. Keep the pressure constant on the inbreath, gradually increase it on each outbreath.

[j.]. Elbows in Top of Leg

Lean into the same point with your right elbow.

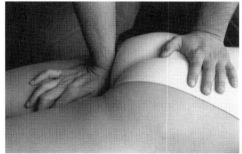

k. Knee Hold

Keep your left hand on the sacrum while you lay your right hand, without pressure, across the back of the knee. Feel how you can hold with your center, even when you're not leaning in with your weight.

[l.] Thumbs down Calf

Lightly slide your right thumb down the midline of the calf a couple inches letting it stop where it wants. The more you stay in your center (instead of going out looking for a point) the more your thumb finds its own way into the points. Let it find its way into the next two points between the two bellies of the calf. Hold each, feeling in your center the oneness of the sacrum under your mother hand and the point.

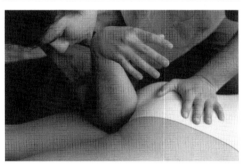

m. Foot Press

Swing up the left foot with your right hand. Up on both knees, lean full weight into the sacrum. This pressure helps protect the lower back while you press down on the foot. Holding the foot just above the toes, gently press the left heel toward the left buttock. Ride over the breath, gradually increasing the stretch with each outbreath (at least three).

n. Far Leg

Lay the leg out straight. Keep your left hand on the sacrum. Lean into the point at the top of the far leg. Lay your right hand across the back of the knee. If you are incorporating work with the thumb, raise your right knee to straddle the near leg and slide your right thumb into three points down the calf. With both knees on the floor, swing the right foot up. Gradually press the heel toward the right buttock.

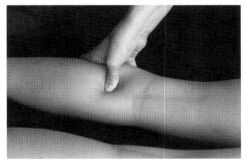

o. Roll Over

Without lowering the leg, slip your right hand to the outside and hold the ankle. With your left hand slide the left arm up alongside the head. Reach across and slide the right arm (palm up) down to the side. Holding the wrist from underneath, pull the right arm up and back, rolling partner over (your right hand pulling, straightening and lowering the right leg). *If you want to finish at this point, do the finish described at the end of this sequence.*

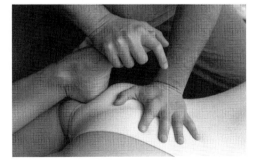

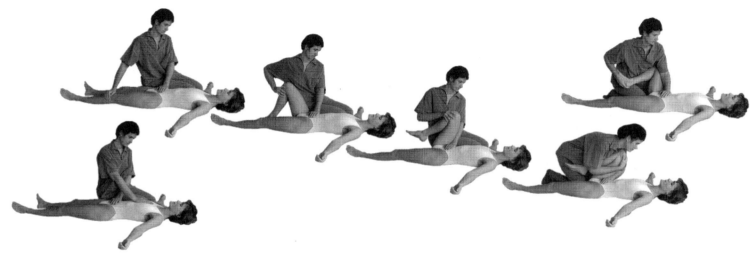

II Leg Cradle

As you cradle and work each leg, one hand stays on the hara body center, a powerful place to 'mother'. As you hold the leg in your lap, feel how you hold it with your Hara. Holding the whole leg this way, helps partner get in touch with its wholeness. Because no part is isolated partner does not know where to resist. Working the leg while holding the hara, helps open up the yin meridians that run up the inside of the leg. We work directly with all three. The connection in this cradle is further enhanced by keeping one knee against the first chakra and the other against the side of the hip.

a. Heart Hara

Partner is lying face up, arms out to the sides. Sit seiza to the right, alongside the hara, your knees toward the arm. Cross your arms, your left reaching across your hara and your right coming from your heart center. Lay your left hand on the Hara and your right on the heart center. Stay three breaths. Feel the connection between these centers, heart and body, the same centers you started from on the other side.

b. The Knees

Keep your left hand on the hara. Slowly lift your right off the heart center. Without changing your position or moving your legs, reach back and rest your right hand on the far knee. Hold three breaths. Place your hand on the near knee. Hold.

c. Leg Wrap

Reach around under the back of the knee. Raise it until the foot is flat on the floor. If needed, lean the knee against your side while you tuck the pants up. Holding the knee from the front, continue raising it until the leg (bent) requires no effort to hold up. Keeping the leg balanced, get up on both knees. Place your right knee on the floor against the first chakra (the perineum, where it stays throughout the sequence,) and your left knee against the outside of the hip. Your left hand still on the hara, drop your left shoulder level with the raised knee. Clasp the bent leg to your chest. Hold it like a baby.

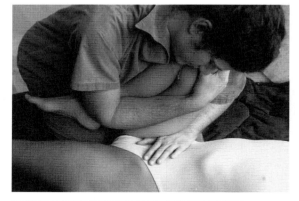

d. Outward Leg Rotation

With your body weight lean the right leg toward the chest slowly stretching it. Keeping it close to your chest, lean it away from the shoulder and continue slowly rotating the leg up to and away from the shoulder. (This is the direction that is less likely to cause any discomfort in the hip joint.) If necessary, adjust your hand on the Hara to keep it from being pressed into the rib cage as you rotate the leg.

e. Foot Rotation

While rotating the leg, slip it under your left arm onto your lap. (Momentarily lift your left hand off the hara if the leg is large.) Sit back on your heels, the leg against your hara. Hold the whole leg with your hara. Without pausing, carry the leg rotation into a foot rotation, rolling your body while clasping the ankle between your thumb and finger (Kidney 6 and Bladder 62) and stretching the foot forward with the pressure of your forearm against its bottom.

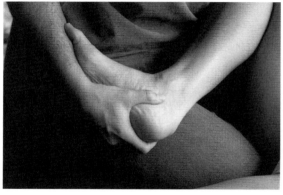

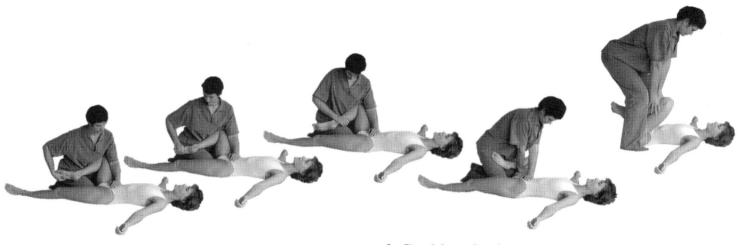

f. Gushing Spring

With your elbow crooked out press your right thumb into Kidney 1 (Gushing Spring) in the bottom of the foot. It is in the hollow in the midline one third of the way from the toes to the heel. Sit with your back straight. Feeling the connection between this point, the chakra in the foot, and the Hara. Hold three breaths. Hold with your hara. . . the stillness that follows movement.

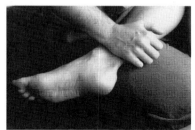

g. Up the Foot

Clasp the foot with a vise like grip, the heel of your right hand pressing the side just below the big toe, your right fingers pressing the other side. Release and reclasp with each outbreath, working your way to and around the heel. Clasp the Achilles tendon.

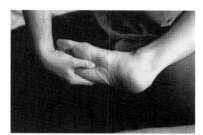

h. Up the Calf

Place the heel of your right hand on Spleen 6 (the Yin Meeting Place) just above the ankle. As you breathe out, rock forward, pressing your heel up under the shin bone, bringing that leg even more into your hara. As you breathe in, straighten up, sliding your heel a couple inches up the leg. Rock forward again with the next outbreath pressing the heel of your hand up under the shin bone. Continue working up the spleen meridian this way until the heel of your hand reaches the knee.

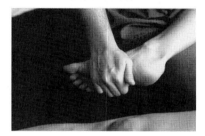

i. Up the Thigh

Place your right hand on the inside of the thigh just above the right knee. Keeping your right knee against the first chakra and your left hand on the hara, rise up. Move your left knee a couple inches away from the hip to give room for the leg to stretch down. Keeping both arms straight, lean into the thigh on the outbreath. As you breathe in, slide your right hand a couple inches further up and lean in again on the next outbreath. Continue leaning into and stretching the Liver meridian until you are near the top of the leg.

j. Knee Press

Take your hand off the hara and hold the right knee, swinging it toward the chest. Take your right hand off the leg and stand, lifting the other knee with that hand. Straddle the bent legs. Hold them with both hands just below the knees (Stomach 36). Keeping centered and relaxed, let your weight press both knees down at an angle that keeps the sacrum flat on the floor, a good stretch for most backs. Hold three breaths.

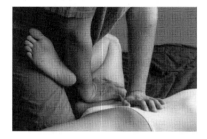

k. Second Leg

Lower the leg you worked on and move to the second side, your knees against the first chakra and hip. Place your right hand on the hara. Clasp the left leg to your chest. Rotate it and do a mirror image of d - j. After pressing both knees to the chest a second time, roll partner to the right, knees up in a fetal position. *When first learning this, if you want to break at this point, instead of rolling partner over, go on to the Finish.*

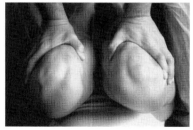

41

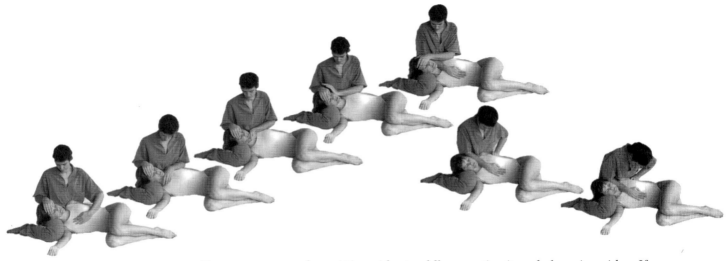

III Back Cradle

If you are not used to sitting side straddle, practice it and changing sides. If your hips are tight, place a cushion under the buttock closest to the floor. If your knee is uncomfortable, try working with one leg straight. As always, adapt and find what works best with your own body. While practicing this cradle, feel your heart and body centers join to hold, move and connect with your partner.

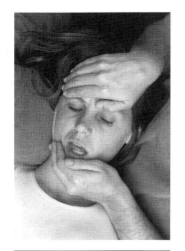

a. Heart Mind

Partner is on the right side, legs up in a fetal position. Have a rolled towel nearby. Face the back, your right leg bent back, your left foot in front, your left toes level with the top of the right shoulder, your left knee against the lower back. Sit as close to your left heel as possible. Simultaneously pick up the left forearm with your left hand and the head with your right hand. While pulling the left arm, slide your right thigh under the head right up against the shoulders. Lay the left arm across your left leg. Without letting the head fall to the side, slip your hand from under the head to over the forehead. Simultaneously place your left hand on the heart chakra. Make sure the head is in line with the body, and turned just enough toward you to facilitate your leg's total support of the neck. Your right hand lies across the forehead, fingers pointed away. It is centered on the third eye. Hold, feeling the connection between heart and mind centers. Straighten your back, feeling the connection in your own body center as you breathe with your partner. Hold three breaths.

b. Chest Corner

Keeping your right hand across the forehead, gently lean your left forearm into the upper corner of the chest on the outbreath. Hold.

c. Chin Open

Keep contact with the chest. Hold and gently move chin to loosen the jaw.

d. Jaw Hold

With your left forearm still on the corner of the chest, fit the heel of your left hand into the hollow under the jaw hinge. Hold lightly without massaging, or moving your hand, which lies gently across the face. Slide your left hand across the forehead to replace your right hand, which crosses under your left arm to lie on the heart center. Hold heart and mind. Focus on the straightness in your back.

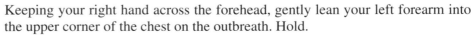

e. Arm

Lift your left hand off the third eye and clasp the upper left arm close to the shoulder. On outbreath, lean over the arm, taking it into your hara, and squeeze. On inbreath straighten your back and slip a couple inches further out the arm. Continue folding your body over the arm with each outbreath. Surrender your back's straightness, and return to it. Continue until your hand squeezes just above the wrist. The whole time your right hand has stayed on the heart center, its pressure never greater than its resting weight.

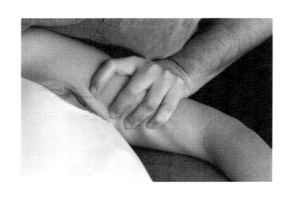

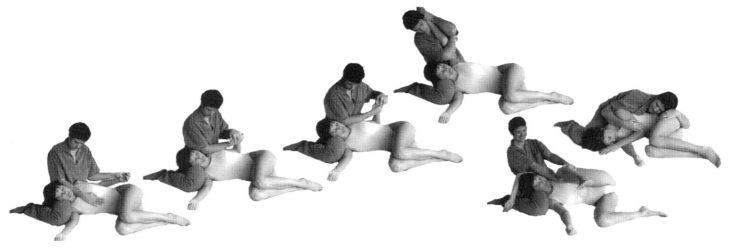

f. Hand Chakra

Hold the center of the palm with your left thumb (without bending the elbow back). Straighten your back. This is the chakra in the hand. Holding this point and the heart center creates a powerful connection. Both are related to the Circulation meridian. Feel the connection in the straightness of your back. . . the stillness that follows movement. Hold three breaths. Sink deeper into your center at the bottom of each breath.

g. Triangle

Move both hands slowly. Your left, holding the left hand, swings the forearm up, the elbow staying on your leg (if possible). At the same time your right hand leaves the heart chakra and catches the wrist of the arm your other hand is swinging up. Your right forearm is leaning across the upper chest, just below the shoulder where the Lung meridian begins. Your forearm and the bent arm form a triangle. With your left hand, gently press down against the back of the hand, stretching it forward. Hold. With your palm over the palm, gently press the hand back. Hold.

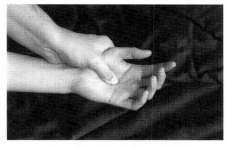

h. Arm Rotation

Hold the left wrist with your left hand, pulling it up to the left of your head. With your upper right arm, hold the arm pressed tightly to your chest. Lean back, stretching the arm. Keeping it close to your chest, holding it like a baby, rotate it by leaning into a circle. Keeping it pulled, change directions as often as you like. It is your upper body, rather than your hands, which is slowly stretching and rotating the arm.

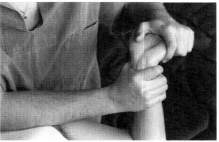

i. Leg Lean

Circling out of a rotation, lay the left arm up over the head. Reach down and slip both hands around the left thigh. Lean back to stretch the leg, keeping the leg close to the side. Hold the leg, your arms straight, letting your body go farther and farther back. Hold. Lower the leg to the front. At the same time reach under and pull the right leg closer to the chest so that both legs are bent up as far as possible into a fetal position.

j. Rest

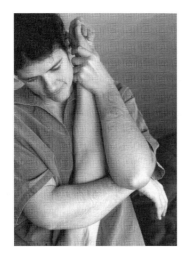

With your right forearm gently slide the left arm, if it is still stretched up over the head, back out in front of partner. As you slide the arm forward, position your right forearm against the top of the left shoulder. Simultaneously move your right thigh just far enough back to let the head slip forward. If partner is very broad shouldered and you think the neck would be uncomfortable, keep the edge of your thigh under the head. This slight movement back of your right thigh is the only change you make in the positioning of your legs. Lie forward and hook your left forearm against the tailbone, resting your left hand on the outside of the leg. Rest your head on the side of the hip. Maintain a constant pressure holding shoulder and tailbone between your arms. At the same time let your chest relax and sink against the back. Feel the connection and stillness in your heart, holding the whole body. Feel how much strength there is in your arms when there is no effort, when you hold with your heart open. Rest.

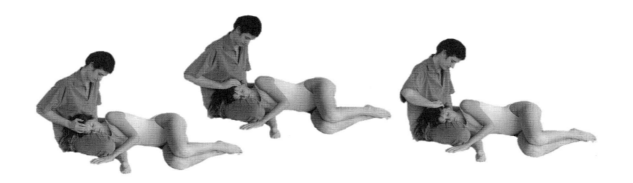

IV Head Cradle

Just as the last cradle encourages us to open and hold more with our heart, in the next we hold and mother someone's head with our body center. This is a position that provides beautiful access to head, neck, shoulders and chest. The more we feel our hands working from our heart when we are holding someone with our body this way, the more we feel how our heart and body are one.

a. Occiput-Third Eye

When you feel the rest at the end of the Head Cradle is complete, straighten your back. Place your left hand on the floor behind you. Slide your right hand under the head and hold it up off the floor. Get up on both knees. Slide your left knee up alongside your right. Switch the head into your left hand and, placing your right hand on the floor, slide your right knee out in front of partner. Sit side straddle with your right foot in front of you, your left leg bent behind you, and lower the head onto your right thigh (the ear between your thigh and your calf). The back of the head is against your hara. Your left knee is against the upper back. Moving into this second side position you have reversed the configuration of your knees without lifting them off the floor. Be sure that you are well above partner so that the neck continues the natural fetal curve of the spine and is not bent back. Hold the large depressions (GB 20) under the occipital ridge to each side of the neck with your left thumb and forefinger. Hold the third eye (just above the nose) with your right middle finger. Sit, enjoying the straightness of your spine. Feel how the points you are holding under the occiput are the backside of the point under your middle finger, feel the oneness in what you're holding.

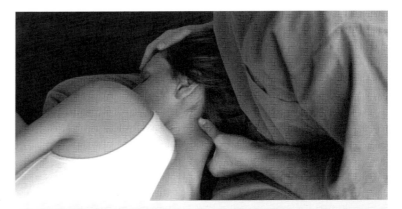

b. Side of Head

Your thumb and fingers still in the occiput, place the four fingers of your right hand on the side of the skull over the ear (not on the temple). As you breathe out, lean forward with your body, feeling how your fingers are finding their way into points in the small hollows and contours of the skull. Straighten as you breathe in, and place your fingers an inch or so further back. Continue, leaning into the skull with each outbreath, working your way toward your thumb under the occiput.

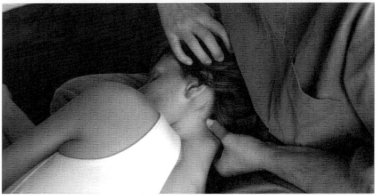

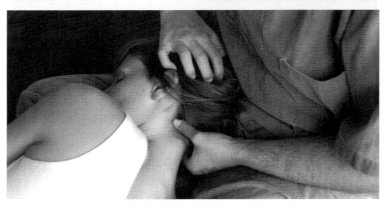

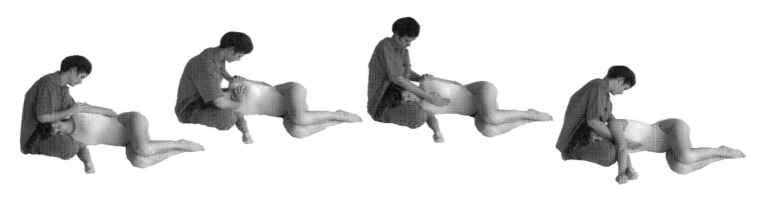

c. Neck

Replace your thumb with your fingers. Hook your right middle finger in the big hollow under the left side of the occiput. Hold with a steady pull while thumb and fingers of your left hand grasp and squeeze down the musculature in the back of the neck. Work down rocking into the neck with the outbreath. Stay with anyplace you feel needs holding. When you reach the base of the neck, start from the top again. The third time you work down leave your left thumb planted in the upper back alongside the shoulder blade (Gall Bladder 21). Hold, feeling the connection between this point and Gall Bladder 20 where your right middle finger is still hooked.

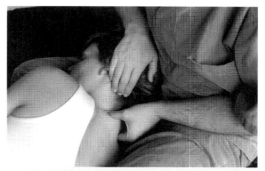

d. Shoulder Blade

Pick up the left arm with your right hand and slip the forearm behind the back. With your right hand pull the shoulder up and toward the front. Place your left thumb under the upper corner. On the outbreath gently slide the blade over your thumb (brace your left elbow on your left thigh). Push the shoulder down and back in a way that keeps the blade open as it slides over your thumb. On the inbreath pull the shoulder up and move your thumb an inch down the edge of the blade. On the next outbreath slide the blade back over your thumb. Repeat until you arrive at the bottom of the blade.

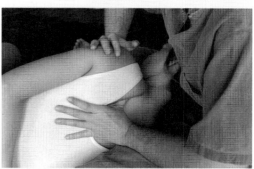

e. Chest

With your left hand pull the upper left arm behind partner to open the chest. Keep it pulled back while your right hand works across the top of the chest. With each outbreath lean your fingertips between the ribs. Work towards and place your right hand on the heart chakra.

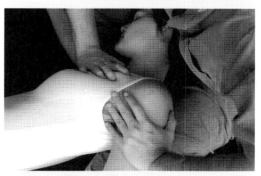

f. Upper Back

Keep your right hand on the heart center as your left lays the arm back out in front. Work down from the neck, on each outbreath leaning your left thumb into the next bladder point (between the vertebrae about an inch to the left of the spine). At the same time gently press the Heart Center, feeling the oneness between your two hands at the bottom of each breath.

g. Heart Hold

When your left thumb arrives behind the Heart Center press the spine with your whole hand. If inflexibility or size do not prevent it, rest your head on the side of the chest, holding the heart center from three sides. Be careful not to put excess pressure on the head which should be comfortably enwombed in your lap. You are holding the two, heart and head, as one. Rest.

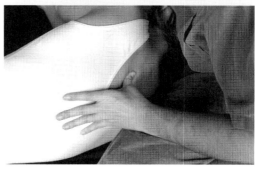

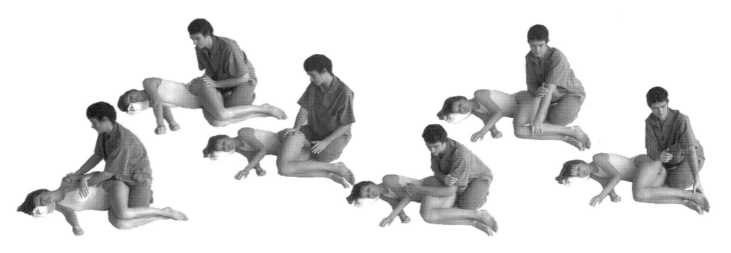

V Hip Cradle

a. Shoulder Roll

Lift the head with your left hand. Slide a rolled towel under it. Pick up the left arm at the wrist with your right hand. Take it with you as you move around the hips. If necessary, push the knees closer to the chest. Up on your knees, straddle and clasp the thighs and lower back. Drape the left wrist over your left arm and firmly clasp the left shoulder with both hands. (Do not interlace your fingers.) Keep the left elbow bent between your two arms by slightly elevating your left arm. Rotate and gently stretch the shoulder, rolling your body and lifting from your knees. Change directions as often as you like. If your partner is too large to straddle the hips at the same time as you rotate the shoulder, start with your knees alongside the back. Adapt.

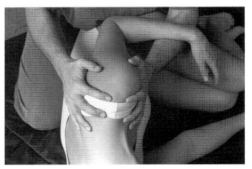

b. Three Speed Hip

Carry the rotation of the shoulder into a rotation of the hip without breaking the flow. Laying the left arm out in front and sitting back on your heels, hold the buttock with both hands and slowly rotate the hip, lifting and rolling with your whole body. Keep your back straight and move partner with just your arms, faster and faster, shaking the whole body free. Place the heel of your right hand in the depression over the hip joint (GB 30) and, keeping your arm straight, vibrate your hand. Lean your right forearm into that depression and your left forearm onto the side of the leg just below the hip. Hold, back straight, in stillness.

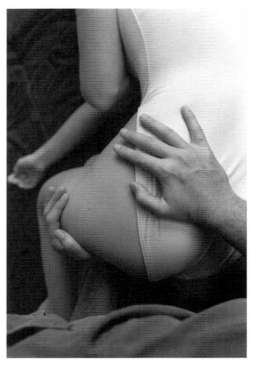

c. Down Side of Leg

Keep your right forearm over the hip joint and, on the outbreaths, gently lean your left forearm into three places down the outside of the left thigh. Continue down the side of the calf with the heel of your left hand, your left arm straight (down the midline, the Gall Bladder meridian, not into the muscle). When you reach the ankle, hold Gall Bladder 40, the depression just in front of the malleolus. Straighten your back and feel the connection between it and Gall Bladder 30, which is still under your forearm. Hold. The Gall Bladder is the meridian of the side. The work we do with this meridian around the side of the head, and under occiput and shoulder blade, culminates in the stillness at this point.

d. Second side

Lay the left arm out to the side. Lifting the knees from underneath, get up on both feet and straddle the legs. With your palms over the calves just below the knees, keeping your back and arms straight, lean in at an angle that presses the knees toward the chest without curving the sacrum off the floor. Keeping the knees bent, roll partner into a fetal position on the left side. Work mirror image of III, IV and V.

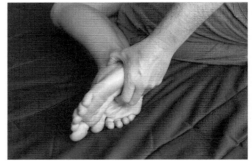

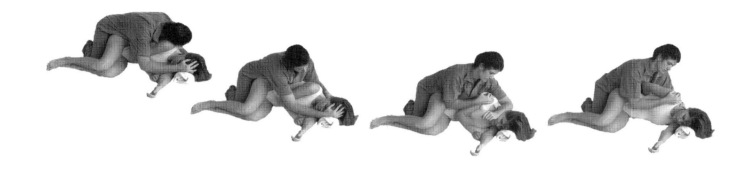

(Cradle of the Second Side)

After repeating the sequence enough to master it, vary the second side by doing it from one position instead of three. Having received the benefits unique to each of the three cradles on the first side, someone can be held in a new way on the second The meridian system is mirrored, and releases effected on one side carry over to the other. It is not necessary to duplicate every move. The first two cradles ended with rests. Begin the second side with a rest. By not doing this side the same way, an element of surprise is maintained. Unlike the other cradles, in which we are partly under a person, in this cradle we lie over them. This is the least size graded and the most encompassing. It is a position that encourages adaptation and creativity. The cradles of the first side culminate in stillness. This one begins in stillness. It is out of stillness that we come into our greatest freedom.

a. Cradle Over

After rolling partner to the second side, slide the towel under the head. The right arm is down in front. Straddle the hips with your legs. Hold the head, the heel of your left hand under the occiput and your right over the third eye and crown. Lay your head on the shoulder and your chest on the side, your body over, or behind, whichever is the most comfortable for both of you. Lie still. Feel the stillness in the holding. Notice what movement is being born in your hands, movement out of stillness. Without looking up, let your right hand be guided over the face and across the side of the head, your fingers pressing in as needed. Free yourself from any need to watch what you are doing. Be with the neck with your left hand. Feel how good it feels to clasp and squeeze the neck, lying still on the side, breathing together.

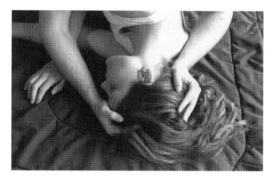

b. Reaching High

Sit up. Up on your knees, still straddling the legs, work the upper torso and arm in whatever order, in whatever way comes to you. You can brace your left elbow on the floor to work your fingertips or thumbs under the shoulder blade. You can pull the shoulder back to work your fingertips across the chest. You can pull it forward to work the upper back. You can pull the shoulder toward you with your left hand while your right holds the arm near the elbow and rotates it. You can pull the arm with your right hand at the wrist, while your left squeezes down, pushing it away from you. You can stretch the wrist back and forth, and work the hand and fingers. Feel free to improvise, but don't feel you have to keep discovering new moves.

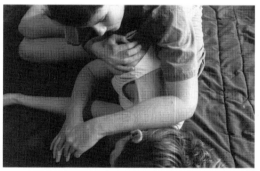

c. Second Leg and Out

Rotate the shoulder and hip and work down the side of the leg as you did in the Hip Cradle on the first side. Lay the right arm out to the back and twist stretch the spine as you did at the end of the first side. If you need to straighten your own legs and get more circulation into them, stand and press the knees down as between the two sides.

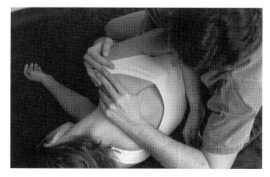

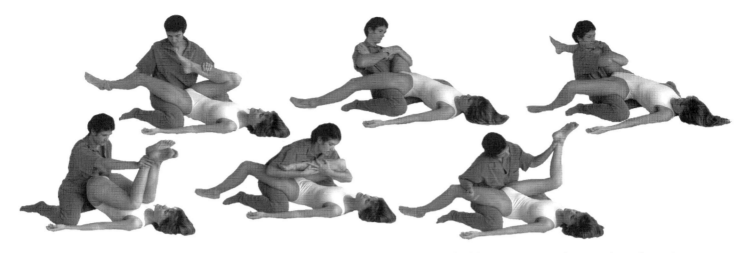

VI Sacrum Cradle

In this final cradle, in which you hold your partner in your lap, there is a powerful connection between the base of their spine and your hara, between their first chakra and your body center. If your partner is too large or inflexible to hold in this position, or if you have any anxiety about its level of intimacy, go directly from the second side to the finish. This cradle is very effective in freeing hip joints and pelvis. It facilitates a lifting roll of hip and leg in a way no other position does. If you want, after doing the first leg, stand up and change the configuration of your legs, but it is not necessary.

a. Leg Roll

Partner is on the back. Up on your knees, push both the calves from behind. As the legs swing up over the head, walk your knees in closer. Cross the left ankle under the right. Hold both with your right hand. Place your left hand on the floor for support. Slide your left calf under the lower back. Bend your right leg out to your side (Side Straddle), and lower the left leg over your right thigh. Clasp the right leg to your chest (the middle of the thigh in the crook of your left elbow, the foot in the crook of your right). Holding the leg close, roll your body to rotate and stretch it. Notice how, when you let yourself lean back, the whole leg lifts, opening the hip. When it is lifted, reposition your calf under the lower back, if necessary. Change directions as often as you like. The leg you are holding supports you, allows you to get your own body freer. It's also something you can rest the side of your head on while rotating. There can be peace in the middle of movement.

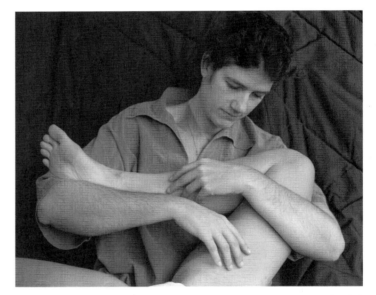

b. Leg Push

Come out of your last rotation pushing the right calf toward the head with your left hand, your left arm straightened. Simultaneously lean your right forearm back onto the left leg just above the knee. Hold.

c. Leg Pull

Without lowering the leg, bend down and catch the back of the right knee over your left shoulder. Clasp the leg close. Making sure the knee does not slip off your shoulder, lean back to stretch.

d. Left Leg

Lay the right leg to your left side. Hold the left leg to your chest and rotate, pull and push as above. Placing both feet on your chest and, leaning into them, raise the sacrum high enough to slip your calf out from under.

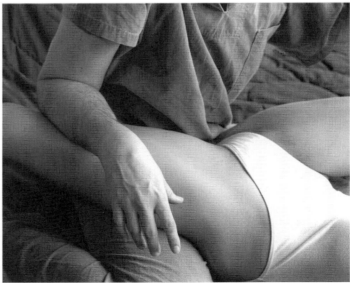

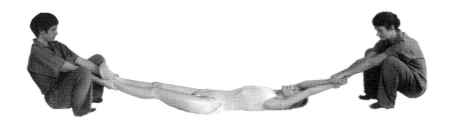

VII Finish

The closeness of the Sacrum Cradle is followed by a stretching out to all sides. Follow the connection and freeing of the lower body by working your way to above the head. Help your partner realize the connection and oneness of the whole body. Many get in touch with the energy that rises up the spine and connects all the chakras. The last places you hold are the heart and mind centers. If you stay still as you hold them and straighten your back, you might feel a rising up your own spine. The sitting that follows your hands' lifting off, can be a powerful meditation. The whole session has been a meditation. You have been working from the emptiness in your center. The stillness at the end of the session, still feeling the connection when you are no longer touching, is the empty in the empty. You may experience sitting at the end a spontaneous vibration up your back. But don't expect it. There can be no anticipation in emptiness, just being.

a. Two Leg Pull

Straighten and hold the legs by the heels. Squat and lean back, your arms straight, your weight pulling both the legs. Lower the feet to the floor, tucking the heels under (toward the head). Lean into the tops of the feet just below the toes, stretching the feet down. Hold.

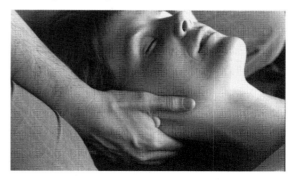

b. Crossed Arm Pull

Stand up and walk along the left side, picking up the left wrist with your right hand. Moving above the head, pick up the right wrist with your left hand. Cross the arms and squat, leaning back with your weight, to pull them. Lay both arms back out to the sides.

c. Head Pull

Sit seiza or cross-legged. Hold the head in your hands. Clasp the skull between the heels of your hands without pressing the ears. Hold under the occiput with the sides of your forefingers. Keeping the neck straight, lean back to pull. Hold.

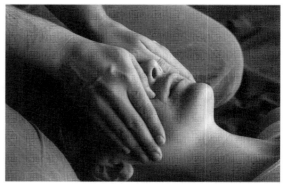

d. Eye Cupping

Straighten your back. Place your hands (fingers outward) on the face, cupped over the eyes (without touching them). Block out all external light. Hold the whole face in your hands.

e. Finish

Simultaneously lay your left hand across the forehead (over the third eye) and your right hand (pointing toward the feet) over the heart chakra. Hold. Feel the balance between these two centers. Feel the straightness of your back, and the energy rising up it. Slowly lift up both hands with the rising. Move about a foot back, but still in line with your partner. Sit. You are no longer touching. Feel in the emptiness in your body center how you are still connected . . . and separate. Be there when your partner is ready to come back.

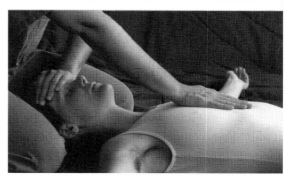

THE HARA

The following sequence on the hara can be incorporated into the Basic Tantsu when you roll your partner onto the back. There are different places during a Watsu where it could be incorporated. First, learn it well on land. Then, include it in your Watsu as suggested in the sixth chapter. Masunaga's says that when we work on someone else we are working on ourselves. This can be particularly felt when we work on the hara.

Ampaku

In Japan, the hara, the area around the center of the body, has an importance, a sacredness, that is echoed throughout the culture and the language. In traditional Japan specialists devoted their lives to working on the hara (Ampaku). Masunaga incorporated Ampaku into Zen Shiatsu. He says work on the hara stimulates the parasympathetic nervous system. This helps normalize the body's basic functions. It calms our sympathetic (fight or flight) system which takes over when we are faced with danger, real or imaginary.

Beginner's hara

Masunaga says the condition of the meridians, their state of balance in the present moment, can be felt, and improved, in the hara. Each meridian has its own area in the hara. The functions of the separate meridians are introduced in the following section. A beginner is better off approaching the Hara with compassion, than with any attempt to conquer and understand intellectually everything that is happening under the hands. If you stay 'empty', while leaning into and holding another's hara, you will feel in your own hara what is happening and what needs to be done.

Precautions

There are certain important reality checks, however. Tell your partner to give you feedback if there is any discomfort. Do not assume your partner will. The whole time you work on the hara watch the face for any signs of distress. Do not work on the Hara after a meal, or when a person has any inflammation or problem in this area, or when their bladder is full. Go slowly into each area on an outbreath. With your right hand extended and relaxed so that it bows backward as you lean in, gently lean in with the parts of your fingers just below the tips. Follow the breath down, feeling the letting go in your own hara. If that letting go feels incomplete, ride over the next inbreath without increasing or decreasing pressure and lean a little deeper on the next outbreath. Continue until you feel the completion, the emptiness, in your own hara. Whenever you feel a pulse, slowly back off. The aorta coming down from the heart should not be pressed into, as there is a danger of its walls being thin. This work, which can be very powerful, often puts people into a deep state of peace.

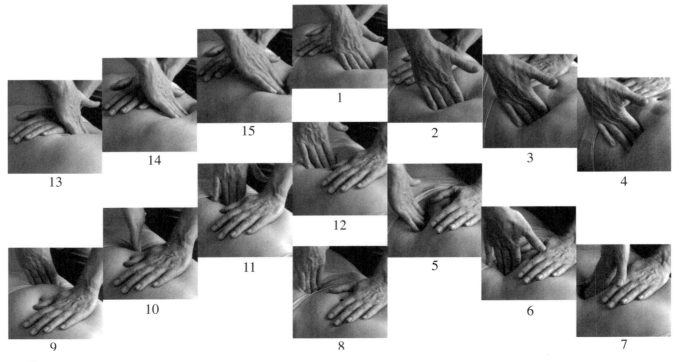

13 14 15 1 2 3 4
9 10 11 12 5 6 7
8

a. The Hara Rock

Sit seiza alongside the hara (to the right). Partner is lying on the back, arms are out to the sides. Neck and head are in line with the body. Cross your left hand onto the hara (from your hara) just below the navel, and your right hand onto the heart chakra (from your heart). Connect to the breathing. Hold at least three breaths. Lay both hands flat on the hara (they shouldn't be crossing the midline and they shouldn't be so close to either the ribs or the pelvis that they pull skin when you lean in). Gently and slowly rocking in from your own hara with each outbreath, cup your hands down and in toward the center. Watch the face for any signs of discomfort. Continue for several breaths.

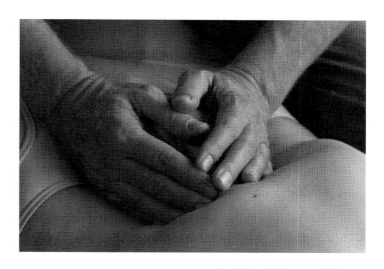

b. The Upper Hara

Place your left hand across the hara under the navel to mother as the extended fingers of your right hand lean slowly on the outbreath into the area of the Heart meridian under the xiphoid process (1). (If you feel any pulse, release your pressure.) Rock back to vertical as you breathe in, your arm slowly withdrawing. On subsequent outbreaths lean into the Stomach(2), Triple Heater(3) and Lung(4), areas which are evenly spaced under the left rib cage.

c. The First 'H'

Slide your mother hand over the Circulation(C) area just up from the navel. With your right palm facing the left iliac spine, lean your fingers into the Kidney(5) area a couple inches to the left of the navel. Turn your hand at a right angle (the crossbar of the H) and lean into the Small Intestine(6) area. Turn it at another right angle (the second side of the H) and with your palm facing the navel, lean into the Large Intestine(7) area under the iliac spine. After making this letter H, return to the midline and lean into the Bladder(8) area just above the pubic bone.

d. The Second 'H'

Make the same H in reverse order, starting at the iliac spine, on the near side of the hara(9, 10, 11). Make both sides of this H with your palm facing away from the navel. Return to the midline and lean into the Spleen Meridian area(12) an inch below the navel.

e. The Return to the Upper

Slide your left hand back down to mother below the navel. Lean into each of the three areas under the right side of the rib cage in the orderP: Lung(13), Liver(14) and Gall Bladder(15). Return and lean again into Heart(1) where you began your circle of the hara (and the spiral into its center). Lay your right hand on the Heart chakra. Hold.

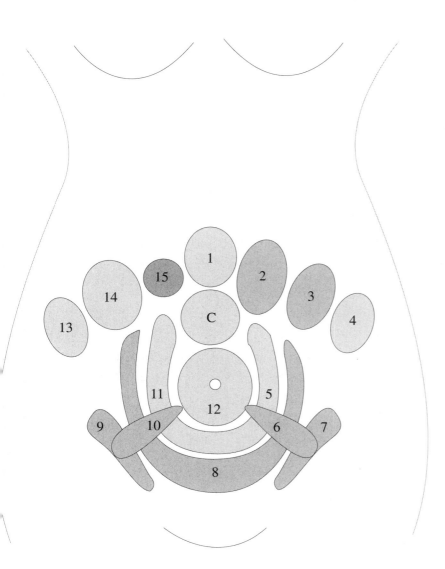

Tantsu and Watsu with Groups

Water Circles

Watsu can be integrated into any kind of workshop or intensive that focuses on personal growth. Practicing Watsu's simplest moves can be very powerful in itself, particularly if you work with a variety of people. Have the participants do the Watsu Round described on page 122. This can be followed in a subsequent session by teaching the Opening, the Basic Moves, and the Closing. The pool can also be the occasion of spontaneous group play and circles, circles that move between joy and stillness. A flattened circle turning allows you to look into the eyes of each person as they pass in front of you. An even tighter circle is created by the person at the end of a line linked by hands turning, winding everyone around him. One way to end circles is by having everyone sink to the bottom.

Co-centering

On land many parts of the Basic Tantsu sequence can be integrated. If it is not a bodywork class, the emphasis can be on experiencing the positions and their nurturing power rather than on trying to learn the sequences. The Co-Centering is the simplest to introduce and will be of value to all kinds of groups.

Circle Tantsu

If it is a group that is focusing on issues of intimacy or Tantra, and a single session is to be devoted to Tantsu, the first of the Basic Tantsu side positions is ideal. With a large group, first explain and demonstrate the moves, and make sure everybody in the group can get into the positions. (Those who will need a cushion to support their left hip should have it nearby. Those who aren't comfortable in this position can just be receivers, or can be shown co-centering to practice on each other in a different part of the building.) Have everybody (which must be an even number including yourself) stand in a circle holding hands. Have the people to each side of you, and every second person around the circle, lie on their right sides in a fetal position facing the center. Those who are giving the Tantsu can imitate you in positioning their left leg against their partner's back and their right bent behind them. Before taking up their partner's head and arm, if the circle is not too spread out, the circle of givers can clasp each other's arms or hands. Then they can simultaneously pick up their partner's arm and head and follow you in all the moves of the Back Cradle from the Heart Mind to the Rest (being part of the circle yourself, everyone around it can see you and be seen). Any assistants you have may walk around the outside of the circle checking positions and moves. On completion, the givers can straighten their backs and reconnect their arms in a circle. When their partners are ready, they can turn over and give the givers feedback. Everyone can stand in the circle again, holding hands in silence. Those who worked (except you) lie in fetus and the others follow your moves. If a second session is scheduled, the full Head Cradle can be done with those in fetal position lying with their feet in the center like spokes of a wheel. A third session could be done with their heads in the center. The Hip Cradle can be immediately followed by rolling them onto their backs and doing the Sacrum Cradle, after which, to be able to finish above their heads, the givers can slide them out a ways by pulling their feet. After they pull the arms and finish, all those who gave can sit back at the center of the circle supporting each other's backs. It is my experience that this work in circles can be very powerful for reinforcing the bonding of a group. It can be a very powerful meditation, a realization of the tangibility of our oneness, particularly for those of us who enjoy feeling it in our bodies. If it is a couple's group, emphasize how, besides helping strengthen the bond of the couple, this kind of work can strengthen a relationship by providing both of them a way to share non-sexually this kind of energy with others.

Bodywork Tantra

Besides the bodywork of this book, its Movement Meditations can be a valuable adjunct to any kind of group. An additional process that works with circles of eight to twelve people is included at the back of my *Bodywork Tantra*.

CHAPTER V

REBONDING THE BODY

When the body is not one

The bodywork in this book is a form of Rebonding. It helps rebonds us to our oneness, the oneness within our body. The loss of that oneness can manifest in either collapse or holding. In collapse there is a loss of tone, of energy, a sense of falling apart. In holding there is tension, a trying to hold ourselves together. Either can be global, affecting the whole body, or partial. Often there is collapse in one part or system of our body and holding in another, a condition which perpetuates the wound of separation in our body. The less oneness we feel, the more we seek it outside ourselves. Seeking in others what we miss within throws us off center.

Holding

If we take refuge in a closed belief system it disconnects us from the spontaneous, nurturing life within. The less connected we feel, the more we feel the need to hold ourselves together. Holding appears in tightened, hardened connective tissue and muscle, in shallow breathing and lungs not allowed to open fully, in sluggish digestion, in constipation, in constricted capillaries and high blood pressure, in restricted movement, in blocked energy and in closed hearts and minds. If we truly and joyfully felt and lived our unity within and without, none of these conditions, and related health problems, would plague us.

Getting in touch with what heals

Rebonding helps us get in touch with our own healing energies. The relaxation it induces loosens holding. The oneness arrived at lessens the likelihood of holding re-emerging. The possibilities of spontaneous creative movement it opens provide a way to continue to access and celebrate that oneness in our body. In addition there are specific ways that Watsu and Tantsu reduce muscular tension, open breathing and lower blood pressure. The most immediate effects are in the musculature. More than anything it is our connective tissue, particularly our muscles, tendons and ligaments, that hold us together, and hold us up. They are the first to tighten. They are the most common places for us to hold the memory of trauma.

Holding in pain

Places where we pull back from pain become places where we hold in pain. Places where we hold back aggression, restraining an impulse to strike or kick out, become places where we hold back all feeling. This holding affects the surrounding area, as antagonist muscles in turn tighten in an effort to restore balance. The relaxation and stretching of Rebonding Bodywork help release these stored tensions and make available to us the energy spent in holding them. Our work with the breath helps deepen the breathing and increase the supply of oxygen to all parts of the body. The warm water and the bodywork lessen the capillaries' constriction and help normalize blood pressure, which in turn reduces the load on the heart.

THE BODY SEPARATED

The disconnected

The more we have the idea, the fear, that our body is not complete in itself, that it is not a unity, that it will on some level fall apart if we do not make efforts to hold it together, the more likely we are to experience separations in the body. The mind is so powerful it can isolate any part of the body and make it feel disconnected, separate from the rest. The most common victims of this in our puritan based culture have been the sexual organs. Each culture creates its own anatomy. In France, the liver is in center stage and blamed for a variety of conditions. In Germany it is the circulation. Each individual takes the body image provided by his culture and modifies it according to his own experience and inclination. The only way to break this image's hold over us is to rediscover the freedom of the whole body and the way its own creative movement comes from within.

Ways we separate

Besides separating out parts of the body, it is common to separate the body into two opposed parts such as left side\right side, front\back, inside\outside, or top\bottom. The latter separation underlies the expressions above the waist and below the waist. It also underlies the concept of someone being too much in their head, though there the separation is seen through the neck. The waist and the neck are the most common places to separate the body into three. In such a three-part separation, each part has its own interior space or cavity defined by the skull, the chest and the abdomen. Our goal is not to separate the body but to find its essential unity. Looking at how it is most commonly separated, and how there are similar unifying principles within each of these three areas, will help us understand how it is unified.

In water

Vertebrates in water, where there is an equal pressure from all sides, tend to have a more obviously unified structure than those on land, who stand up under the pressure of gravity. When a fish moves, its whole body moves in wave motions that propel it through the water. There is no separation of the head from the rest of the body. Their spines are very flexible. In the new born this flexibility of the spine and unity of movement can be seen. When a baby cries, its whole body cries. We carry in our bodies memories of all the stages of both our individual development and our development as a species. In Watsu, in its wave like movement of our spine, we return to that aquatic stage and its unity.

On all fours

In animals who move on all fours, there is a clearer separation between the limbs that move them and the rest of the body they are moving, but that doesn't prevent them from moving in total unity, as when a tiger springs. It is just a more complicated unity than that which the fish moves in. For humans, getting down on all fours and letting our bodies move freely, gets us in touch with a level of basic emotions associated with the second stage of our development.

Upright

In the third stage, which is that of our rise into an upright position, there is a clear separation between the nature and functions of our lower and upper limbs. This is reflected in the differentiation the Chinese make between the energy in the three pairs of meridians that flow through the arms and the three that flow through the legs. Their energy, in turn, is differentiated from the energy in the central meridians which relate to the spine and the head in our upright position.

In this third stage the way to unity is even more complicated than that of the springing tiger.

The Way to Unity

Expressing the freedom of the whole

The way we breathe, the way we move, the way energy flows through us, the way we make love, are among the many ways we have been given to know our unity and honor the divine within us. Each of these, and every part of our being, has its own dynamic, its own freedom, its own way of expressing the freedom of the whole. When that expression is denied, each becomes as much victim and victimizer as individuals in a totalitarian state, a state where conflict and tension replace the love that holds us together.

The Loving Breath

The breath's freedom

Given its freedom, the breath enters every part of our being with love. Since it can only be free when it's free of conscious control, it is difficult to approach the breath, to become conscious of it, without compromising its freedom. Learning to do this is the basis of many meditation techniques. Letting our body sink and rise naturally with the breath is the most basic technique of Watsu. The more we can be with our breath this way, the more we can be with others in a Rebonding session without needing to control what is happening.

The void

There is the breath that fills and the breath that empties. Between the filling and the emptying, there is a moment of total fullness. Between the emptying and the filling there is a moment of total emptiness. This emptiness we sink into at the bottom of the breath is the void we experience in our meditations. It is the void out of which the creation that each breath creates rises.

Resistance

Those parts of our body where there is holding resist opening to the breath. This fear reappears in our inability to completely let go at the bottom of the breath. Releasing tension helps those parts open to the fullness of the breath and helps us let go into that creative void.

The breath within

At times, in the stillness of a Rebonding session, we enter back into that void and, without interfering, feel how every part of our body opens and welcomes the rising breath's loving caress. During a Watsu the feeling of the breath filling our body can be as delicious a feeling as the warmth of the water on our body's whole surface.

Moving from Freedom to Freedom

The music we dance to

Being open to the breath is a precondition for freeing the spontaneous loving movement that can be initiated by any part of our body. On this level the breath is the music our bodies dance to. A simple experiment will demonstrate this. Hold your arm out to the side. While holding your breath, move your arm. Now keep your arm held out there with as little effort as possible. Breathe naturally and deeply and let your arm move however it wants. Notice how, the more you let this happen spontaneously, the more the movement will spread down your side and through your body. How much more unifying and free, moving this way becomes than when trying to move while holding the breath.

Habit's waste

Restricting our body's movements to those established by habit, or to those initiated by our will for specific purposes, denies our body its freedom. Through disuse much of our body's potential can be wasted and lost. Denying our body the neurological information and challenges of unique spontaneous movement accelerates its aging. The wound of separation increases as we become alienated from what our bodies can do.

Neurological information

In Watsu, as we discover the spontaneity of movement in our own body, and move someone more and more spontaneously through the water, we are showing them how good it feels to let their body move in unique, uncontrolled ways. The Creative Movement Meditations of Rebonding Therapy encourage them to approach their own body with a love that does not feel threatened by, but delights in its freedom.

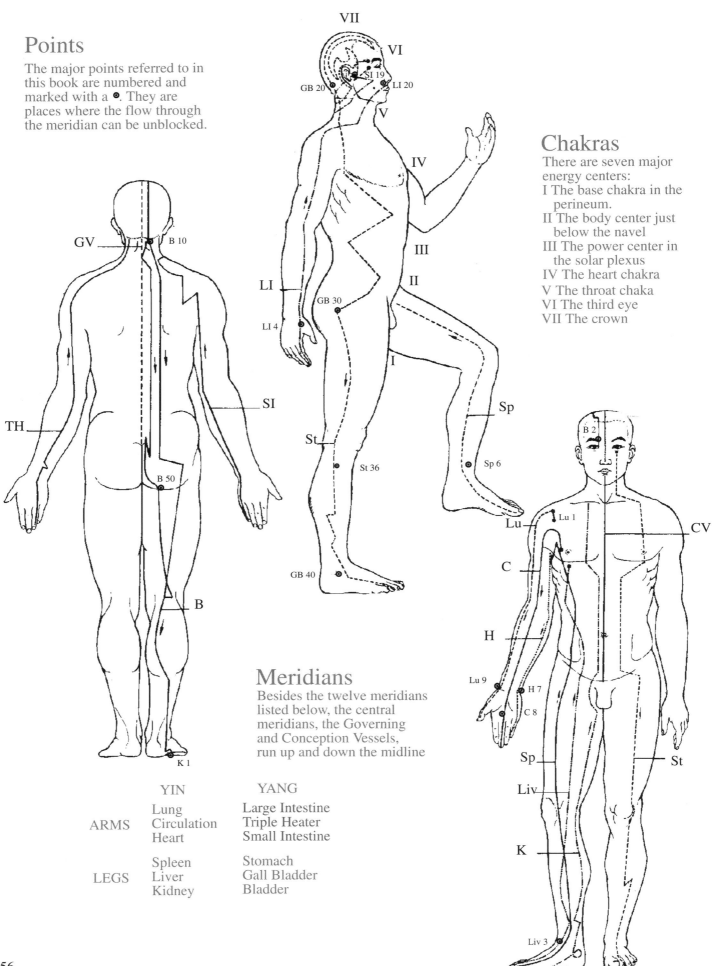

Points

The major points referred to in this book are numbered and marked with a ⊙. They are places where the flow through the meridian can be unblocked.

Chakras

There are seven major energy centers:
I The base chakra in the perineum.
II The body center just below the navel
III The power center in the solar plexus
IV The heart chakra
V The throat chaka
VI The third eye
VII The crown

Meridians

Besides the twelve meridians listed below, the central meridians, the Governing and Conception Vessels, run up and down the midline

	YIN	YANG
ARMS	Lung Circulation Heart	Large Intestine Triple Heater Small Intestine
LEGS	Spleen Liver Kidney	Stomach Gall Bladder Bladder

GV
B 10
TH
SI
B 50
B
K 1

VII
VI
SI 19
GB 20
LI 20
V
IV
III
II
LI
GB 30
LI 4
I
Sp
St
St 36
Sp 6
Lu
GB 40

B 2
Lu 1
CV
C
H
Lu 9
H 7
C 8
Sp
St
Liv
K
Liv 3

THE ENERGY CONNECTING

The breath is to the inside of the body what movement is to the outside. Both have a clearly defined object to which they are related; whereas energy, by definition, exists outside time and space. There is no limit to the ways energy can pour into, rise up, flow through, wheel around our bodies. There is no single theory that can contain all its manifestations because it is, if anything, creative. To try to contain it inevitably leads to dualism, to naming that which cannot be contained as nonexistent or evil. In Rebonding we stay as lovingly open to it as to our freed breath and the movements originating in our body. We dance to it. Watsu often moves into a pure dance of energy.

The Points

Clustering around the joints

There are points on our body where energy tends to become blocked (and where it can be released). Most of those that acupuncture classifies as major points cluster in or near the body's joints. In ideal health the chi energy in our bodies would be in continual motion. It would never meet any resistance. The nearest approach to this ideal state is when the body is in water. Once we step out of the water there is resistance. The joints and the muscles attached to them need to hold the body in fixed positions. Our bio-energy concentrates in these points to perform this task. Because of physical or emotional trauma, it over concentrates in certain points. At first this over concentration, this tension, is an excess of energy in the point that can be released easily with the appropriate movement and/or pressure. But over time, if it is not released, the energy concentrated there can become atrophied and no longer accessible, in which case the acupuncturist or bodyworker's task is to gradually bring more energy through this point from that released elsewhere in the body.

Kyo and jitsu

Acupuncture and Shiatsu classifies the meridians and their points as either in excess or depletion (Jitsu and Kyo in Japanese), that is in states of holding or collapse. In the west, the points are referred to as trigger points and their locations are confirmed by the sensitivity in them being relieved by extended pressure.

The Meridians

The life force divided by functions

The meridians are pathways of energy that connect the points. In *Zen Shiatsu* Shizuto Masunaga emphasizes that stretching Meridians (Chi Kung in China) is even more ancient than the work on points done in acupuncture. Mammals, on waking, stretch to mobilize their energy. Masunaga says the Chi that flows through these meridians is our 'life force' and the meridians are the functional division of that life force. Each meridian is where the flow of energy related to a particular life maintaining function is strongest. These are common to all life, even that of a single cell. Where the meridian appears on the body relates to its particular function. Stretching a meridian brings it closer to the surface and helps open up its energy without having to go painfully deep into those points along it where chi tends to become blocked.

Yin and yang

Traditionally meridians come in pairs. In each connected pair there is a Yin and a Yang Meridian. Where the energy flows from one into the other is at the extremities of our arms and legs. The Yang end of each pair is in the head (The three that extend down the legs start around the eyes). The Yin end of each pair is in the chest around the heart. If someone stands with their arms up, the flow of the energy in the Yang meridians is from heaven to earth, and the flow in the Yin from earth to heaven. In the fetal position the Yang meridians are those which are on the outside exposed parts of the body.

Stretching

There are stretches for each meridian that help them return to balance. In Watsu it is not necessary to methodically stretch meridian after meridian because all the meridians will get stretched many times over during a session. Being stretched spontaneously while the whole body is being moved makes it more difficult for the recipient to mobilize habitual resistance. Neither is it necessary to diagnose which points are Kyo or Jitsu and treat them in any special way, nor to ask a person which points are sensitive. The stretching and the rocking continually work the joints freer and freer, releasing energy blocked in all of them. Given enough stimulation, our body's own self healing mechanism will respond and complete any balancing begun in Rebonding bodywork.

Knowing our own body

Our knowledge of the points and the other forms of energy is based on their presence in our own body. While working with someone, when we feel our oneness with them, we should trust our intuition and hold whatever places feel they need to be held. The more we are in touch with these forms in our own body, the more our intuition will guide us to them in others. The following lists the major points on each meridian. These are the points that have the farthest reaching effects. Find and get to know each of these on your own body. For more detailed descriptions of these, and the rest of the points, consult one of the many available books on acupuncture. The stretches included in the Movement Meditations presented later in the book will also help you get to know the different forms of energy in your body.

Connection to the Earth

Front

It is with our legs we stand on the earth. The legs and their energies do not stop at the hip joint, but are very much connected into the pelvis and the abdomen. Masunaga describes the function of each of the leg's three meridian pairs as related to where they appear on the body. The three pairs are the meridians of our front, the meridians of our sides and the meridians of our back. The meridians of the front, the stomach and the spleen\pancreas, are at the front of our body because we go out in front of ourselves to get food. They are related to the earth element. The earth is where our food grows. The strength that comes from food is governed by these meridians. Excessive energy in these meridians could be reflected in tendencies to be always going out in front of ourselves, in obsessive thinking, etc. The earth element is also connected to the area around the navel, to our physical center. We center and ground ourselves in the earth. Whenever we press the foot toward the buttock, or move a person through the water as the leg is pushed back, we are stretching and opening the stomach meridian. Stretches which turn the partially extended leg outward open the Spleen meridian. The most powerful point on the stomach meridian is Stomach 36 just below the knee. The most powerful on the spleen meridian is Spleen 6 above the ankle.

- Stomach 36. *Three miles of the Feet*. Besides strengthening the legs to walk long distances, this point is used in acupuncture for almost every condition.
- Spleen 6. *The Crossing of the Three yins*. The three Yin meridians of the legs cross at this point which is used for all female conditions. Avoid during pregnancy.

Sides

The meridians of the side are the Gall Bladder and Liver meridians. The Gall Bladder Meridian flows down the outside of the leg and the liver up the inside. Masunaga describes their positioning as having to do with making decisions- "Which way to go, to this side ... or to this." Whereas the Stomach and Spleen meridians have to do with our strength, and its source in our food, these meridians have to do with how we use that strength, with our power. When our power, when our ability to make decisions is thwarted, the emotion associated with these meridians can come to the fore, which is anger. The time of life associated with these is Birth. The element is wood, wood when it is green growing out of the earth. Twisting or stretching one leg across the other opens the Gall Bladder meridian. Pressing the bent leg outward and up opens the Liver meridian. The Gall Bladder's major points in the leg are Gall Bladder 30 and 40. The liver's is Liver 3 in the foot.

- Gall Bladder 30. *Bouncing Ring.* Effects conditions in the hips and legs.
- Gall Bladder 40. *Hilly City.* Normalizes Gall Bladder Meridian.
- Liver 3. *Big Rush.* For abdominal cramps and emotional instability. Induces abortion.

Back   Whereas the above two pairs have to do with the strength we get from the earth and how we use it, the third pair, the Bladder and the Kidney meridians, have to do with how we return it to the earth, with our elimination, which is the recycling, the purification of our energy. Their element is water which returns to the earth. Their color is black. Their time of life is death, which is a return to the earth. These are the meridians of the back, of what we leave behind. And what we don't leave behind we carry on our back. Each meridian has its own area along the bladder meridian where what is not let go of in those separate meridians ends up on our back. The lowest of these areas is the sacrum, which relates to the bladder meridian itself. When we bring the legs toward the chest we are stretching the Bladder and Kidney meridians. A powerful bladder point on the leg is bladder 50 just at its top. The most powerful Kidney point is Kidney 1 in the bottom of the foot.

- Bladder 50. *Receive Assistance.* For sciatica and paralysis of the lower members.
- Kidney 1. *Gushing Spring.* For Kidney problems, heart pain, high blood pressure, Coughing, irritable children, sterile women, coma, shock, hysteria and epilepsy.

Connection to others

Outside   Just as the legs and their meridians' functions are closely related to the abdomen, the arms and their meridians are related to our chest and the lungs and heart contained within it. Our legs are what stand and walk over the earth, our arms are what reach out to hold those we love . . . or push away those we need to push away to establish our boundaries. The Lung and Large Intestine meridians are the meridians of the outside. Masunaga describes their function as the interchange between the inside and the outside. They have to do with our boundaries. The skin is related to these meridians, as is the nose, speech and grief. Their element is metal as transformation and their color is white. Their Major points are:

- Lung 1. *Central Palace.* For cough, asthma and facial edema.
- Lung 9. *Large Deep.* Balances Lung Meridian.
- Large Intestine 4. *Meeting of Valleys.* Affects teeth, throat, face and hand.

Inside   The remaining two pairs of meridians in the arms are both related to the element fire. The meridians of the inside, the Heart and Small Intestine, whose function is assimilation, relate to our innermost fire, to our deepest, most personal center, the heart-mind. This is the center of our feelings and our love. This is where we are most personally vulnerable. The function of our meridians of the surface, the Circulation and Triple Heater meridians, is the protection of this deepest center. Both this surface fire and our innermost fire are expressed in joy and laughter. The tongue and sweat relate to them. Their major points are:

- Heart 1. *Extremely Important Spring.* For conditions of heart, chest and upper arm.
- Heart 7. *Gate of Gods.* Balances heart energy.
- Circulation 8. *Palace of Labor.* Effects circulatory conditions, shyness.

Speech   That the meridians of the arms are related to the tongue and speech, points up the connection between our hands and communication. Our hands' role in our connecting with others is not limited to touch and holding, but extends into our spoken communication where their activity is in direct proportion to the intensity of our communication. The speech of people who 'sit on their hands' is more separated from their deeper being and reaches us less deeply than someone who is speaking from their heart and their whole body.

Connection to Heaven

Freeing the spine

Whereas the legs and the arms relate more to the second and third stages of development, the spine dates from the first. Though it has lost much of the flexibility it originally had in water, when we feel in it what flexibility it is still capable of, we are closest to our aquatic nature. In Watsu's continual wave like movement, the spine becomes freer and freer, so free that there can occur a spontaneous rising of energy up it.

Microcosmic circuit

The central meridians, the Governing Vessel that rises up the spine, and the Conception Vessel down the front, are channels of energy in a stage more complete than the twelve meridians. It is the Lake of Heaven out of which the twelve flow. The Yang of the rising kundalini up the spine and the Yin of the slow settling down the front is a contrast, a counter flow to the Yang and the Yin in the twelve meridians. In Taoism this is the microcosmic circuit, a microcosm of creation. Our chakras, which are described below are closely connected to this cycle.

Base of the skull

All twelve meridians are represented by areas and points alongside the spine. Between each process there is a point on the Bladder meridian an inch to an inch and a half alongside the spine. At both ends of the spine are major points. Those under the occiput effect most conditions related to the head, including vision. They are:

- Bladder 10. *Pillar of the Sky.* Affects head and neck.
- Gall Bladder 20. *Windy Pool.* For common cold, headache, stiff neck, hypertension.

Face

There are major points around the eyes, at the base of the nose and in the Jaw hinge. The points in the face and head effect primarily what is most immediate to them. They are:

- Bladder 2. *Gathering Bamboo.* Affects head, eyes and face.
- Large Intestine 20. *Welcoming Fragrance.* For nose and sinus.
- Small Intestine 19. *Palace of Music.* Affects ear.

Connecting it all Together

The more we feel the connection of all the parts within each of the three regions described above, the more we can feel how they are all connected together.

Sex unifying

Just as restricted movement and breath can turn something that has power to unify into something that separates, so can our love life when it comes from a separated space. Though the sexual organs are located in the lower third, they can have a powerful connection to both the heart and that which rises up the spine. Their power to unify is unlimited, but when they are suppressed as less moral or spiritual than other parts, when they have been abused and traumatized by the warped sexuality of others, they are deep in the wound of separation. Sexual wounds, and the fear of them, affects our ability to open up to any form of intimacy.

Sex separating

Separated and vulnerable, our sexuality, often finds itself being used to help fulfill the functions of one or more of our meridian pairs. For many the primary use of sex is to release tension, a form of elimination not unlike the others that are the function of the Bladder and Kidney meridians. Functions of other meridians of the legs are implicated if we use sex to ground, to enter the earth, to prove our strength or power, to dominate. The meridians of the arms can be involved in using sex to connect to others or to establish boundaries.

Tantra

Sex's potential to unify is best realized when we open to the central meridians, the microcosmic circuit that runs through our sexual organs. In Tantra connecting to this flow up the spine and its opening of the heart as it settles back down the front becomes a powerful spiritual practice, a spiritual practice that is no way based on downgrading or separating out any part of our being. The more we experience this totality of creation present in each of us, in all our being, the freer we are of the duality that creates such spiritual havoc, such separation in our lives.

THE CREATION CYCLE
AND THE CHAKRAS

Resonating   Whereas the energy in the meridians is in a state of flow, and the points are where that flow has blocked, the energy in each chakra is a completeness, a unity. This has been described as the whirling of a circle or spiral. In the meridians the energy moves from one point to another. In the chakras the energy resonates, its resonance connecting it to our other chakras and the chakras of others in a way that is a loving unity. But even here, in looking at, in systematizing these most unifying forces of our being, duality can creep into classifying them as higher and lower, as denser and more refined. The antidote to this tendency is to feel how total each chakra is. If, at the bottom of the breath, you let yourself sink completely into the first chakra, you will experience the emptiness, the void out of which all creation comes. There is nothing more total than this. This is the Tao, the undifferentiated, the mother of all beings.

In the *Tao Te Ching,* Lao Tzu says,

> The Tao gives birth to the One
> The One gives birth to the Two
> The Two gives birth to the Three
> And the Three to the Ten Thousand

What we feel rising up the back is the Tao giving birth to the One. The One is our crown chakra, where we are one with everything, a place of light. My own most powerful experience of this was rising up into what I had seen as a city of light and suddenly being the light, being its shining out to all sides, no longer seeing but being light. This rising up the back is followed by a settling down the front, an emptying back into the void, a return to the Tao which is continuously giving birth to the One. This is a continuous cycle. Where we can feel this continuity most is at the center of that cycle, midway between the rising and the settling, midway between the Tao and the One, in our innermost heart center, which is our most personal, most vulnerable place. That center and the center in our head, our innermost mind center, are the Two that are born out of the One, the Yin and the Yang, Heart and Mind, Soul and Spirit. These are the two poles of our meridian pairs which create and maintain the life of our body. Our body has its own center on the surface just below the navel, and the heart has a center on the surface, and the mind at the third eye. These are the Three we face the world with: body, heart and mind, our strength, our love and our clarity. Between these are the centers in the solar plexus and the throat- the center of our will, our action, our deeds; and the center of our communication, our words. Our deeds and words are the Ten Thousand that are born out of the Three.

Experiencing   Reading about chakras is no substitute for experiencing them. Both the giving and the
chakras   receiving of Rebonding open and harmonize these centers, particularly the Heart chakra. Another center that opens more in Rebonding than in other forms of bodywork is the first chakra in the perineum. The non-sexual support it receives, particularly in Watsu and Tantsu when people straddle our leg or our waist, is a powerful aid in getting people in touch with the microcosmic circuit, and the creation cycle of which the first chakra is the base. At the end of this book you will find meditations that guide you through this creation cycle and its return, the emptying of everything back into the Tao. Experiencing how the whole of creation is present in your own body is Rebonding.

On Being in Rebonding

Spiritual practice

Rebonding is experiential. It is being with the experience, being with another, being with whatever happens. It is Rebonding to that part of our being which experiences directly, freeing ourselves from those parts that direct or interpret our experience. That part in which we are one with our experience is that part in which we are one with everything. This everything includes those parts that direct and interpret. They have their place. Creation would be impossible without them. But to the degree they keep us from being with our experience, they perpetuate the wound of separation. Rebonding is a spiritual practice. It is not a religion. It is not a system of beliefs. No one is told to believe anything, just to be with whatever they are experiencing. Any attempt to interpret or diagnose, to read another's aura or chakras, to channel guidance, to tell another what is wrong with them, or what they should do or believe, is contrary to the spirit of Rebonding. If we set ourselves up as the one who knows, we distance ourselves. If the person we practice with looks upon us as a doctor or a shaman or a guru, etc., they replace the immediacy of experience with their habitual dependancy on authority.

Observer self

This is not to say we should repress our natural tendencies to direct and interpret. Whatever is repressed finds its own secret, sometimes more damaging, way to exert itself. It is better to be aware of every part of our being and its place. Developing this awareness, this observer self, is essential to all spiritual practices. Be aware of whatever part of your being resists being in the immediacy of an experience. Accept that part into your awareness. Be aware of whatever part comes in after an experience to interpret it, to try to make it happen again. Accept that part into your awareness. Accepting, giving it a place in your awareness, undermines whatever power it has over your behavior.

On the Place of Belief in Rebonding

During a Rebonding one may move into states of being which have no place in their belief system. Rather than being a threat or a challenge to that system, this should point up the irrelevance belief has to the immediacy of our experience, which calls for a suspension of disbelief not unlike that demanded when reading poetry. This similarity to the esthetic experience, which creates its own immediacy, points up the creative potential in being at one with our experience.

Belief's limit

Shifts of belief can open us up to experiencing in ways we might not have been able to before. But each new belief can, over time, develop into its own closed system. I remember my first contact with the new age doctrine that we create in a succession of lives, situations through which our soul is continually growing. It gave me a new way of looking at, of being with others, respecting whatever they are going through as a creation that has meaning. But over time, if that belief becomes closed into a system that pretends to explain everything, it can close us to the immediacy of the pain that others are suffering. Both a belief in the survival of the soul and a disbelief in it can limit us. An absolute belief in it can cut us off from the sweetness, the uniqueness of the passing moment. Disbelief can close us to the full range of possibilities in a creative universe. Creativity is all around us. All we see and feel is being created, and is itself creating in a way that would be impossible in a closed predetermined universe. I can't imagine a creator with unlimited power being satisfied with creating something closed. It is much more interesting to create a universe like ours where creativity is unleashed. It may be that all our visions and experiences of divine light, our past lives and the tunnel of light filled with friends waiting at the moment of death, are all testimony to how powerful we create in our moment of life. Whether they are still there or not when that moment is extinguished is irrelevant.

Closed systems

Man's tendency to embrace closed systems that try to explain everything is nowhere more apparent than in the systems that have been built up around the energy we feel in and around our bodies. The complexity of these systems is in direct contrast to the phenomena, which when they occur, are as immediate as the fingerprints of God.

CHAPTER VI

EXPANDED FLOW AND VARIATIONS

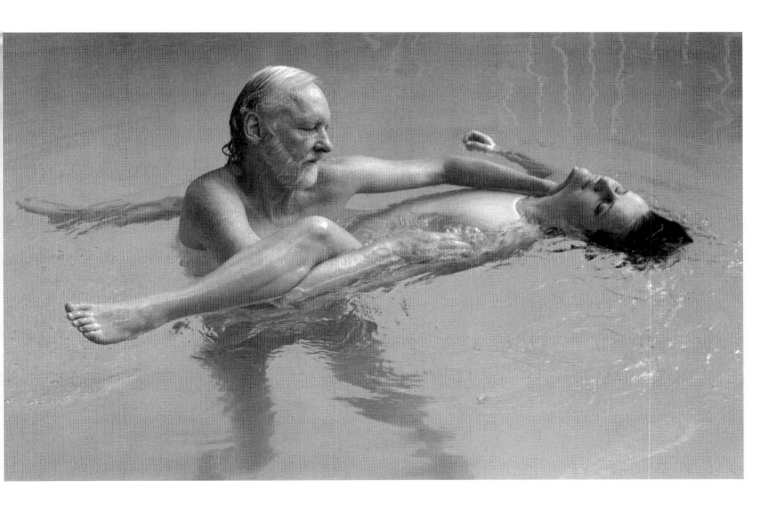

Master thoroughly the Transition Flow and explore on your own the possibilities each position offers, before beginning this chapter.

Expanding the Transition Flow

Additional bodywork that can be done in each of the three sections of the Transition Flow is first presented. Moves which are unchanged from the Transition Flow are titled in Italics. They are preceded by the same letter as when they were first presented. Moves that are numbered are new. An optional fourth section which can be added to the Expanded Flow completes our basic Watsu sequence.

Variations

The next part of this chapter introduces additional expansions and variations that can be incorporated into a Watsu. These, too, are optional, some being size graded (marked with ⊗) and more difficult to execute than moves presented earlier. A sequence that can be done while sitting with someone on steps is also introduced, as well as sequences by Alexander Georgeakopoulos and Elaine Marie. The chapter ends with an introduction to Free Flow.

I Expanding The First Section

The Head Cradle

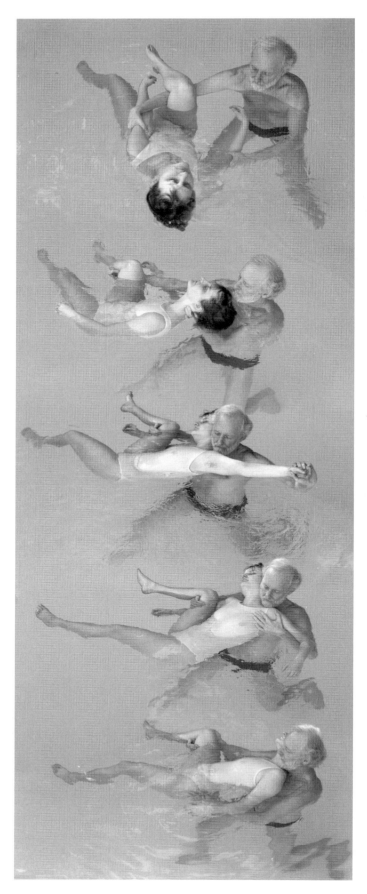

a. Capture or

Variant Capture

Another way of moving someone into the head cradle from the first position is to float them out holding the far arm. During the final basic move, while rotating the near leg up towards the far shoulder, your right arm under the knee, take hold of the upper left arm with your right hand. Float your partner away from you, sliding your left arm out from under the neck. With your left hand take the right arm out from behind your back and place it between you. Hold the head in your left hand. Let go of the left arm and slide your arm along the back of the knee until the heel of your right hand is fitted between the tendons in the back of the right knee. Keep hold of the knee with your right hand while you lower your right shoulder under the head. The right arm should still be under your right arm. With practice, this can be done as one uninterrupted move.

b. Arm Leg Rock.

1. Arm Leg Rock II

After rocking someone from side to side, alternately pulling the right knee and the left arm, you can create a more intense rock by not letting up on the pull to the opposite side. That is, you can keep both knee and arm pulled, and turn your whole body from side to side. This, too, can be done to your breath.

2. Arm Opening

Hold the upper left arm with your left hand. Squeeze, shake and slowly work down to the left hand, freeing the whole arm. Hold the hand and pull it up and back over the head, stretching the whole body by pulling the right knee at the same time.

3. Chest Opening

Reach under the left arm and hook your fingers into the upper corner of the chest. Pull back to stretch the chest open.

4. Shoulder Rotation

Hold firmly above the shoulder joint and rotate the whole left shoulder with your left hand.

5. Shoulder Blade

Place your thumb between the upper back and the shoulder blade. Lifting your thumb rhythmically, work down the inside of the blade.

6. Bladder Meridian

Work down the line of points (bladder meridian) between the vertebrae, an inch to an inch and a half to the left of the midline of the spine. Hold each point with your left thumb and rock the body into your thumb. Continue down over the sacrum to the point just to the left of the tailbone. Hook your left middle finger into this point and rock.

7. Wall Knee

Still holding the knee, slowly back up to the wall. Straighten your left leg to brace your back against the wall. Bend and lift your right knee up into the lower back (to the right of the spine just above the sacrum). Place your left hand on the hara just below the navel and (a) press down. (Avoid putting pressure against the kidney.) Hold. (b) To lengthen the spine, pull the right knee towards the chest while your knee presses against the top edge of the sacrum (to the right of the spine). (c) Place your knee to the right of the tailbone and push the right leg down.

c. Twist
d. Knee Head Rock
e. Second Side

(Free Float)

f. Stillness
g. Free Movement

8.⊗ Side Change

In the Free Float you can move from side to side by pushing up against the near hip at the same time as you pull the head. Switch hands under the head and, from the other side, push the other hip up as you start back to the first side. If not difficult, repeat several times. The last time, instead of going all the way around to the other side, lay the head over your left shoulder and hold the hips with both hands.

(Under Head)

h. Hip Rock

9. Hara Rise

Place your right hand under the sacrum and your left hand on the hara. Push down with the left hand on the outbreath. Push up with the right hand on the inbreath. Continue for several breaths, making sure the feet do not touch the bottom when you push down. Do not do this move if your hand doesn't reach the sacrum.

10. Buttock Rock

Hold a buttock in each hand, the head still on your left shoulder, and move partner slowly through the water. Move and rock from side to side lifting alternate buttocks. Explore more playful, rapid movement to release tension in buttocks and back. Hold still a moment.

11. Slide up Back

Brace the heel of your right hand against the top edge of the sacrum and slowly slide the heel of your left hand up the lumbar spine lifting vertebra by vertebra. The fingers of your left hand are pointed towards the feet. Stop halfway up the spine and begin again the slide up. Repeat again. This third time continue the slide up the spine to the occiput, turning your hand so your fingers are pointed towards the head, and pull the occiput and sacrum apart, stretching the spine.

12.⊗ Forearm Lift

Hold the occiput and skull with both hands. Pull the head as you lift a forearm between spine and shoulder blade, slowly rolling partner toward opposite side. Lift under other side and roll back. Continue lifting with alternate forearms, your elbows pointing towards the feet, all the while pulling the head through the water, stretching the neck. Come out to the right and slip the right arm behind your back to return to the first position.

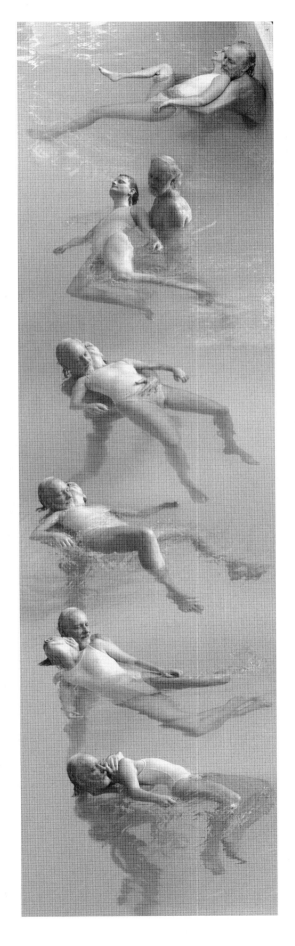

II Expanding the Second Section

a. Far Leg Over
b. Leg Push

1. Down Back

Hold between scapula and spine with your left hand while your right, reaching over the buttock, works Bladder meridian points down the left side of the lower back, sacrum and tailbone, rocking the body into your fingers. Hold Bladder point at the top of the leg firmly with your right thumb and rock partner from head to toe. Still holding the upper back with your left hand, push the right leg out again. Turn in the direction the water's resistance helps stretch the leg back.

2. Foot

Pull your stomach in and bend the right leg so that its lower half lies across your hara below your navel, the right foot in your right hand. Make a pincer with your thumb and finger to hold the ankle while rotating and stretching the foot with your forearm. Hold Kidney 1 (in the midline one third of the way down from the toes) with your right thumb. Work the foot freestyle.

c. Sacrum Pull

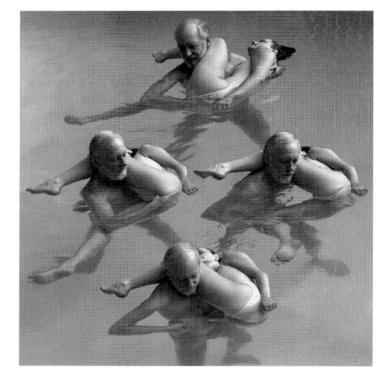

(Under Shoulder)

d. Under Shoulder
e. Lengthening Spine

3. Twist Over

After pushing the sacrum up, reach over the near leg and under the far knee. Pull the far leg across while your other hand holds down the left shoulder. Gradually twist stretch spine.

4. Figure Eight

Let go of the left knee. Quickly reach under the near leg. Take hold of the far leg just above the ankle. Pull it under the near leg and up to the surface. As the hip rotates back, pull (don't push) the leg all the way under to the other side. Repeatedly inscribe this figure eight. Keep your left elbow raised enough to prevent the neck from being strained back.

5. Lower Back

Let go of the left leg when you have pulled it farthest under the near leg. Before partner lays back, press your forearm into the side of the lower back turned towards you. Rocking partner with your forearm, continue pressing between the sacrum and the rib cage. Put no pressure on the spine.

(Under Hip)

f. Spine Pull
g. Undulating Spine

6. Thigh Rock

Reach over the near leg and, holding the buttock with your left hand, clasp the left thigh tight to your waist. Keep hold of the occiput and skull with your right hand. Rhythmically turn away from partner so that your body tugs and rocks the thigh clasped to your side, releasing tension in the near hip.

7. Bow

Reach under the near thigh and over the far thigh to hold the middle of the far thigh in your left hand. Brace the bottom of the buttocks against your side and pull the far leg back, gently arching the whole body.

8. ⊗ Lift

If partner is not too heavy or inflexible to lift out of the water, slip your upper left arm under both knees. Bring them up to the chest as you clasp the upper far arm with your left hand. Pull partner up, the near arm still over your right shoulder, the side of the buttock propped on your hip. Stand high enough out of the water to allow the head to fall forward, without the nose going under, and release any tension lying back in the water might have built up in the neck. Hold the upper right arm loosely in your left hand. If easily accessible, work the neck with your right hand. While still upright, slip your right arm over the left arm and lower partner back into the first position (still on the second side).

9. Neck Pull

If you are right handed, you will find you have your stronger arm cradling the neck when you are in the first position on the second side. Brace your left forearm against the top of the spine while pulling and working the neck with your right arm.

Second Side

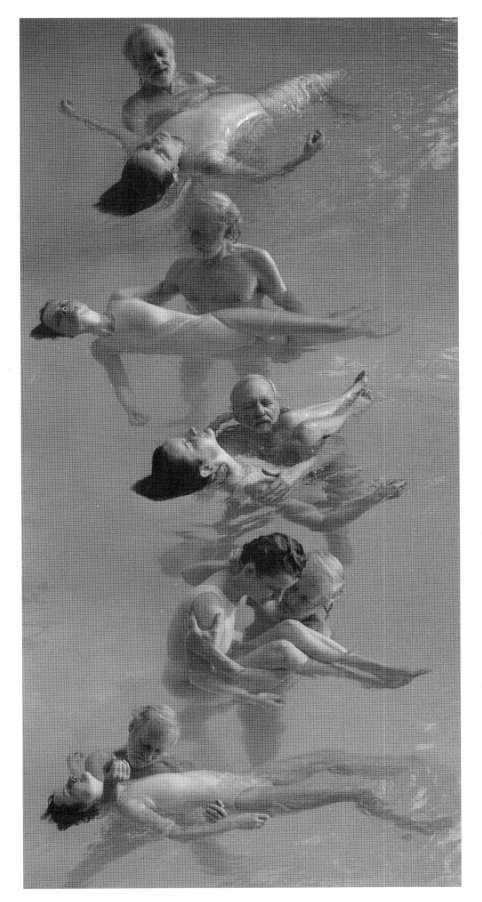

III Expanding The Third Section

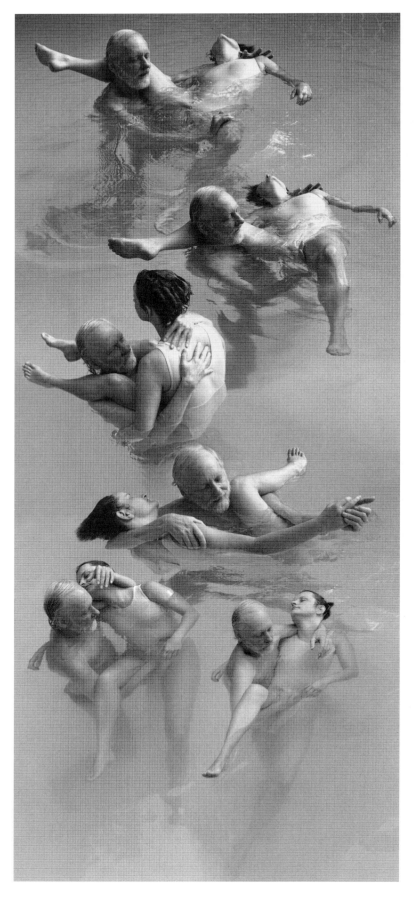

a. Near Leg Over
b. Down Quads

1. Up Liver

After working down quads to below the knee, press the heel of your right hand against the inside of the thigh just up from the knee. Pushing to keep the stretch constant, rock the leg as you gradually work up the inside of the thigh (Liver meridian).

2. Down Bladder

Just below the buttock, press your right thumb up in the back of the leg. Repeatedly lifting with your thumb, slowly work the midline down the back of thigh, knee and calf (Bladder meridian). Turn, pushing the far leg away from you.

c. Leg Down or

⊗ Variant- Both Knees Over

With the near leg over your shoulder you can drape the other leg over your other shoulder and swing your partner up (from the side) into a vertical position. Press the upper back towards you with one hand and work the neck with the other. If you want to use this as a transition from one side to the other, you can lower partner to opposite side and push out the leg you haven't worked yet. If you are in a shallow pool, this might be an easier transition from side to side than pushing the leg down.

d. Leg Pass
e. Arm

3. Freeing the Arm

Free the arm. Squeeze, shake and move it freely. Your right hand can stay in one place, squeezing, mothering, the upper arm (or left shoulder if your arm is not long enough to reach under the neck to the arm). Work wrist, hand and fingers free. Tug the left thigh with your left arm to slip the right leg off your shoulder. Return to position 1.

f. Second side
g. Heart Home

4. Hara Rock

Slide your right hand down to just below the navel. Clasp the hara between your thumb and fingers. Rock. Gently squeeze the hara each time partner breathes out. (If not readily apparent, place your ear close to the mouth to hear/feel the breath.). Gently tug, pull, the hara with each inbreath.

5. ⊗ Hara Spiral

While rocking, circle the hara with your extended but relaxed fingers and gently press into the meridian areas in the way described at the end of the fourth chapter. Do not press into any area where you feel a strong pulse or there is discomfort.

ADDING A FOURTH SECTION

The following has three parts, any one of which can be incorporated by itself into your Basic Watsu. Each is optional. In A we capture a person on our hip. In B we set them facing us on our leg. Both place us on a higher level of non-sexual intimacy because of the contact with the person's first chakra in the perineum when they straddle our waist or our leg. Whenever you feel you might be uncomfortable with this contact leave A and B out of your session. Another situation in which it would be advisable to leave out A would be if you are watsuing an inflexible 'sinker' with a weak neck who is bigger than you. B and C have to be left out when you are in water without any wall to lean back against, or if the water is too deep for you to brace yourself against the wall. You can first learn these in the order C,B,A and then put them together A,B,C.

A. The Hip Cradle

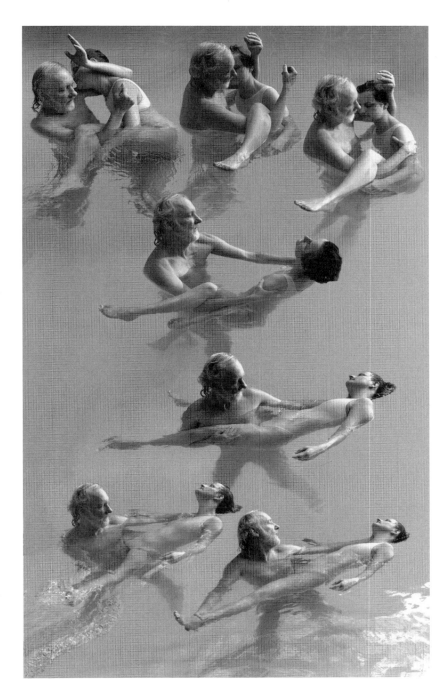

1. Leg Lift
Repeat the Basic Moves. Rotate the far leg. While rotating it, move the body in such a way that you can clamp the near leg between your thighs. Hold that leg clamped and with your right elbow lift up under the left knee to stretch the left leg at the same time as your left arm lifts the torso into a more vertical position.

2. Hip Capture
With your right arm still under the raised left leg, grab hold of the upper left arm with your right hand. Holding the neck with your left hand (over the shoulder), step between the legs. Face the leg you are holding and let go of the arm. By lifting under the knee with your right arm raise partner closer to the surface, and over your left hip, to straddle the left side of your waist. Let partner lie as far back in the water as you can without straining your arm still holding the neck

3. Leg Tug
With your right arm that was under the knee, hold the left thigh from underneath and tug firmly.

4. Leg Rock
Leaning back against the right leg, rhythmically push the extended left leg out in front of you.

5. Leg Pull
Still holding the occiput in your left hand, with your right hold the left leg as close to the foot as possible. Open your arms stretching the whole body. If partner is too tall for you to straighten the torso, focus on pulling, lengthening the leg.

6. Foot Press

With your right hand hold the top of the left foot near the toes and, bending the knee, slowly press the heel towards the left buttock.

7.⊗ Foot Prop

Staying low in the water, prop the left foot (the knee still bent) across the very top of your left leg (or your right, if partner is not flexible enough to prop over your left). Reach under the upper back with your right hand and hold partner up at an angle that keeps the foot against your leg. (If the water is too deep for you, you may need to put one foot up on a step to keep the foot propped). With the leg the foot is not propped on behind you, rock forward and back in whatever way best keeps the foot propped. While still rocking work down the left side of the spine hooking the fingers of your right hand into the bladder meridian. Hook those fingers over the top of the left shoulder. Hold and rock. (If you can't keep the foot propped, work down the left side of the spine. Transfer hands under the head and, without stopping to work on the face, work down the right side.)

8. Face

Keeping the neck and head comfortably held in your left hand, with your right hand work freestyle the left side of the face and scalp. Slide your right hand under your left and hold the neck with both hands, the head raised. Keep holding partner with just your right hand while your left works the right side of the face and scalp.

9. Second Leg

With your left arm reach under the right thigh and lift partner up over your right hip causing the propped foot to go free behind you. Work a mirror image of the above moves (3 - 7). After working the shoulder, reach down with your left hand and move the right foot away from you. At the same time, with your right hand lift the head and settle it comfortably on your left shoulder.

B. The Wall Cradle

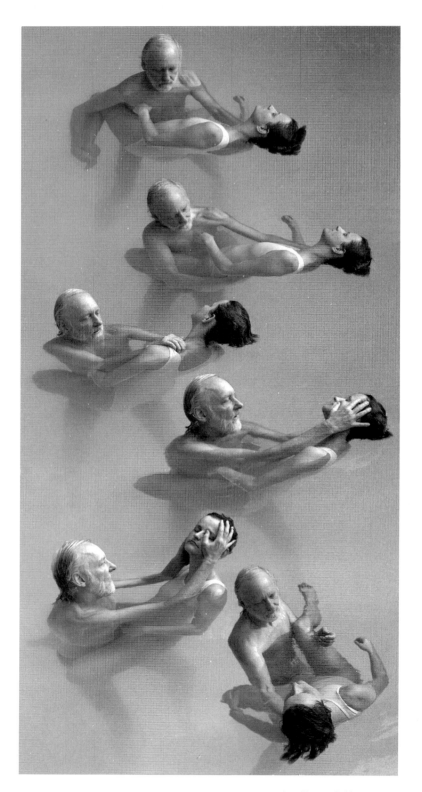

1. Straddle.

Back up to the wall, the head comfortable on your left shoulder, the right foot in your left hand. If you are not coming from the hip cradle, you can roll partner up into this from position 1. Approach the wall carefully so that the head doesn't collide against it. Your right leg, straightened out, helps you brace your back against the wall. Your left leg lifts to the inside of partner's left leg and bends at the knee as you prop your left foot over your right knee. (In shallow water you may find it more comfortable crossing your left shin over your right shin.) If you are coming from the Hip Cradle, let go of the right foot. Partner should be comfortably straddling your left thigh and knee, chest against your chest, abdomen out a ways from yours. Hold the upper back with four fingers to each side of the spine.

2. Back Press

As partner breathes out, breathe out pressing the fingertips of both hands into the upper back. Continue working down both sides of the spine (bladder meridian), simultaneously pressing the fingers of both hands into points with each outbreath. After holding the last points beside the tailbone, press into the hip joints from both sides.

3. Up Back

Pressing your fingertips into the hip joints begin slow circular movements with both hands. Gradually increase the rate of circling as you work up to the lower back. Work up both sides of the spine with small rapid circling. Carry the circling up into the area of the right shoulder between the neck and the scapula.

4. Shoulder Work

Work the right shoulder with your fingertips. Place your right thumb under the upper corner of the scapula. Hold the shoulder with your left hand and, on the outbreath, slide the blade over your thumb. On the inbreath pull the shoulder back forward and place your thumb an inch or so lower. Continue, sliding the blade over on each outbreath. When you have worked down to the bottom of the blade, clasp the shoulder between the heels of both hands and rotate it.

5. Arm Back

Place the right arm (bent) behind partner's back. Squeeze the upper right arm with your left hand while your right hand slowly squeezes down the arm. Press the right palm with the heel of your right hand pushing the back of the hand into the left lower back.

6. Arm Rotation

With your left hand hold the right forearm just past the elbow and, bracing the scapula with the heel of your right hand, rotate the arm up towards, and out from, the head.

7. Twist Across

Come out of the rotation slipping the arm between you (level with your navel). With your right hand pull the right wrist out to your right side while your left hand reaches behind the neck and pulls the left shoulder back to gradually twist stretch the now vertical spine. You may need to use your left elbow, or your own head, to help keep the neck straight. Put the head on your right shoulder and return the right arm back out to the right side.

8. Second Side

Holding the right hip with your left hand, move partner onto your right leg. Prop your right foot on your left knee and do a mirror image of the above (moves 4. - 7). After returning the left arm to the left side at the end of the twist, let partner rest still against your heart center a moment.

9. ⊗ Uncradling

With your left hand thread the right arm between you and start pulling the wrist with your right hand as if you were starting the first twist again. When the left leg is just about to slip off your right knee, let go of the right wrist and pull the knee up to the chest with your right hand, bringing the back against your chest. Switch hands under the pulled up knee and pull the right knee up to the chest with your right hand. Pull both knees to the chest stretching the lower back.

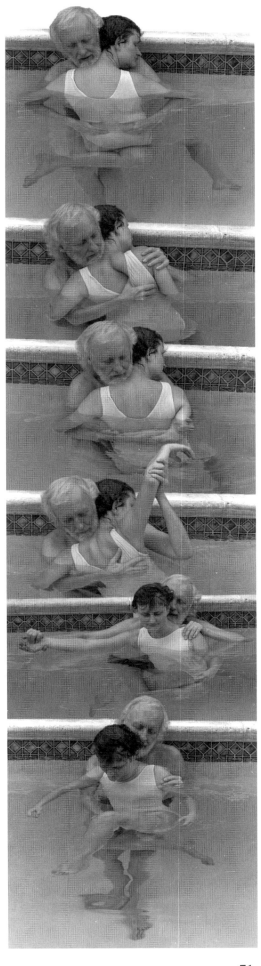

C. The Wall From Behind

If you are coming from the Wall Cradle *you already have both knees in your hands. Otherwise you can start from the* Free Float *and, holding the near leg in one hand, move into the* Under Head *position and pull the other knee up. (If you can't reach it, try slowly pushing the extended leg against a wall to bend it into within reach.)*

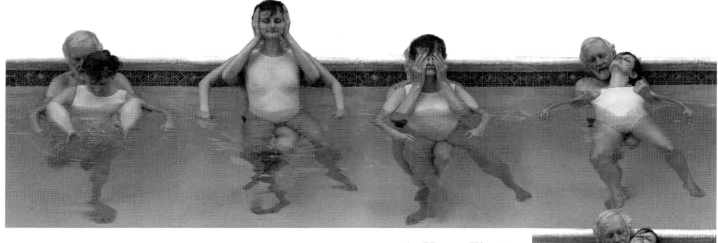

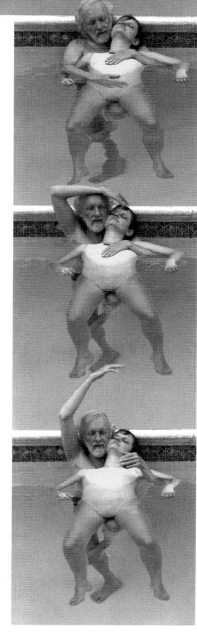

1. Knee Float

With the head on your left shoulder and a leg held just above the knee in each hand, move partner freely around the pool. Alternately rotate each leg.

2. Head Lift

Reaching under the arms, hold the occiput and skull in both hands and pull through the water. Back up against the wall and, using your legs to lift you up, lift the head up vertically to stretch the neck. While still lifting, bend and raise your left knee. Lower partner down (still vertical) onto your left thigh (straddling your leg), your left foot braced against your right leg.

3. Face Work

Lean your forehead against the back of the head. With your arms reaching up under the shoulders, hold the jaw hinges with the heels of your hands, and as much of the face as your hands comfortably cover. Work freestyle with both hands. Hold over the eyes to block all exterior light. Your thumbs can also work points under the base of the occiput.

4.⊗ Chest Opening

Hold the head and gently bounce your knee working partner out into a horizontal position that is as close to the surface as is comfortable, the tailbone on your left knee. Lay the head on your left shoulder without letting it stretch too far back or touch the wall behind you. Still reaching from under the arms, hold the upper corners of the chest with both hands and pull open the chest.

5.⊗ Heart-Hara

Keeping your left arm under the arm, lay your left hand on the heart center. Reach your right arm over the right arm and lay your hand on the hara just below the navel. Hold, feeling the connection between these two centers.

6.⊗ Third Eye

Keeping your left hand on the heart center, slowly lift your right off the hara. Shake your fingers to remove excess water. With your middle finger slide up the top of the nose to the third eye. Hold. Focus on your spine and what you feel rising up it. With that feeling of rising, slowly raise both hands up high. Lower them to under your partner's hands. Hold the hands to the surface, your middle fingers under the middle of the palms. Slide the head out your left arm and, reaching down with your left hand, move the right arm behind your back. Float out in position 1 and finish.

FURTHER EXPANSIONS AND VARIANTS

The Opening and The Completion

In a pool with no wall   If you are in a pool that doesn't have walls to lean against, you can either start standing in the middle or, if there is a ledge, start with partner lying on it. Standing, you can start from either the side or from behind. Stand to the right side. With the right arm behind your back, hold the heart center from both sides. Lean partner back into the first position.

Starting from behind   An alternative way to start, is to stand behind and let partner lean back against your heart center as, reaching under the arms, you pull back the shoulders to open the chest. When you step to the right side, and slip the right arm behind your back, you will arrive at the first position. A more dramatic variation of this is to have the person facing the wall. Pull both arms straight back as you slide down the spine with your right foot slowly bringing partner to the surface.

Finish without a wall   When there is no wall, or when someone is too limp to lean against it, you can end by sitting someone on the steps. If there is no wall and no steps, you can end by pulling them up onto the shore, if there is one.

Final sweep   When someone is leaning against the wall, or sitting on the steps, you can follow the removal of physical contact with moving your hands in such a way that currents of water sweep over their whole body and gradually recede.

The Basic Moves

Variations in first position   Each time you return to the Basic Moves between sections, feel free to explore variations. In this first position, most variations arise out of how we use our right arm and/or how we use our body. Explore the different ways you can hold someone with your right arm while your left is under the neck. Explore how reaching over the body to hold the opposite side varies the way you can hold and move someone. Explore how, when your hand is under the sacrum, alternately standing higher out of the water, letting them turn away from you, and lowering yourself into the water, turning them up towards you, puts their spine through a slow rolling twist. If they are flexible enough, as you lower yourself, you can bring them right up over your right shoulder, and hold them there a moment.

Shake and swing   When you have your forearms under their neck and sacrum, hands down, find the shake or movement of your own hips that best carries a syncopated movement through your arms into their spine. When you have your arm under the knees, stand with one foot out in front of you. Find the forward and back movement of your own body that best starts their body swinging out and back. Explore the shallower parts of the pool to see if there are ways to momentarily set them on your knees or prop them against your body to add support and stretch.

Standing twist   A simple, but effective, twist-stretch can be added while rotating the near leg. Just as you did with the near leg at the beginning of the fourth section, capture the far leg between your thighs. With your left hand push the right shoulder away, while your right pulls the left shoulder.

Massaging   You can also vary how you use your hands by introducing the kinds of strokes, muscle kneading and brushes found in massage. This can be more effective if you have floaters under the neck and the limbs to free both of your hands. But such a set up could compromise the nurturing derived from Watsu's closeness.

Expanding Section IV

This can come at the end of the fourth section's first part with people who do not have lower back or neck problems.

1.⊗ Back Lift

Determine, before beginning a session, that someone is comfortable floating without having the head supported. At the end of the Hip Cradle, after working the second side of back and shoulder, unprop the foot from the top of your leg. Float partner out in front of you, the legs straddling your waist. Move through the water swaying partner from side to side without letting the head hang too far back. If the neck is strong, work the bladder meridian, lifting with both hands down both sides of the spine. Do not lift so hard the head comes out of the water. Remember, the neck is to be treated as that of a newborn.

2.⊗ Double Roll

Do not try this with people who are inflexible, heavy or larger than you, nor with people who have lower back or neck problems. This can follow the above Back Lift. If the head has been hanging back, reach up and stretch the neck to straighten. Hold both feet near the toes and press both heels towards the buttocks. Holding the person slightly out from you, bend the feet in your hands in such a way that they start the bent knees towards the bottom. Staying as low in the water as possible, cause the body to slowly roll up and forward in the water until the head comes to rest on your left shoulder, heart center against your heart center. Still holding both feet in such a way that the lower back is not pulled into too sharp a curve, slowly move through the water. (A variant is to swing partner up with one foot and back up to the wall to do the Wall Cradle.)

3.⊗ Leg Spread

After the Double Roll, with the chest still against your chest and both the feet in your hands, lower the knees towards the bottom. With your knees to the inside of the legs, slowly open your legs, pressing against the insides of the thighs, spreading, stretching the legs apart. Hold the stretch. Let go of the left foot and back up to the wall to do the Wall Cradle.

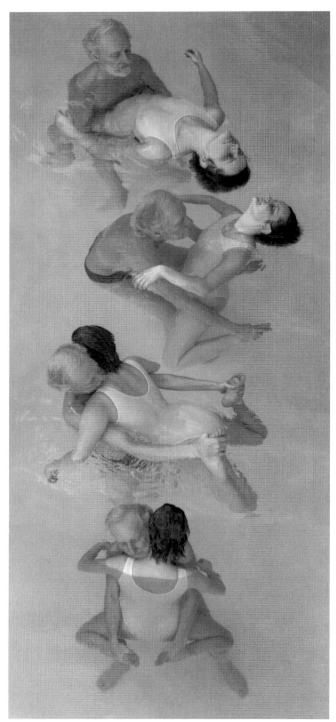

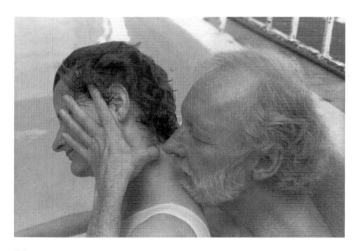

Chin Work

After the Wall Cradle and The Head Lift, set partner on your left leg, your left foot propped over your right knee. Press your chin into the shoulder. Keep one thumb in the largest hollow under the occiput (Gall Bladder 20) on the opposite side of the head, while your other thumb works down the side of the neck to where your chin is placed. Move your chin into the other shoulder and do the mirror image of the above. Lean your third eye against the back of the head and continue with the Face Work.

The Knee Cradle

The Knee Cradle is limited to those who are flexible enough to wrap their arms around the insides of their bent knees. It can be inserted between any of the expanded Watsu's sections. It's best to start from the Free Float position on the second side.

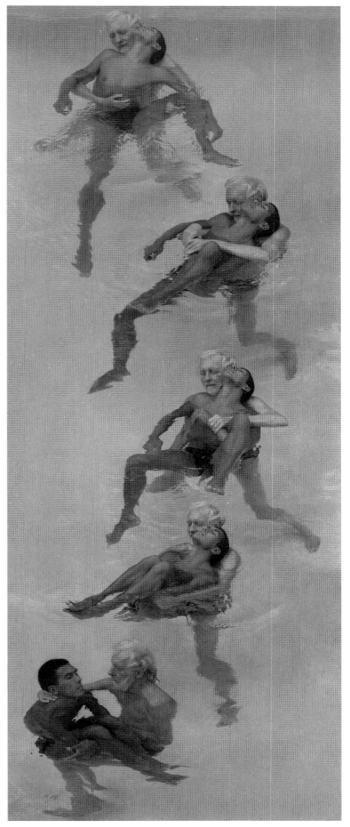

1. Leg Rotation

Reach over your partner's near arm and with the heel of your left hand hold the back of the near knee. Keep hold of that knee as you move behind and, with your right hand place the head against the left side of your chest. This is similar to the 'capture' in the head cradle except, rather than staying low in the water in order to capture the head against your neck, you stand tall in the water to keep the neck as vertical as possible. Bracing partner against you with your right hand on the hara, slowly rotate the left leg up to the chest and away from the shoulder.

2. One Leg Wrap

Hold the left leg to the chest with both hands. With your left hand slip the left arm behind the left knee. Hold the left wrist with your right hand, then with your left hand, the back of the knee locked in the crook of the elbow. Let the head slip onto your upper left arm and, reaching down with your right hand, rotate the right leg.

3.⊗ Two Leg Wrap

Pull the right leg to the chest. Slip it over the left arm and push it against the left leg, pulling the left wrist with your right hand. Hold the left wrist with your left hand (both knees captured over the left forearm) and, with your right hand, push the right forearm under the knees. Hold the right wrist with your left hand and the neck and head with your right hand as partner floats out in front of you (both the forearms under the knees).

4.⊗ Basket Float

Keeping the head well out of the water with your right hand to avoid any feeling of panic that might ensue because both arms are locked under the knees, explore whatever movement this position facilitates. Holding the head and left wrist at constant levels, explore swinging the hips up to the opposite side and back to you. Set partner, turned towards you, on your raised left thigh. The spine is vertical and the buttocks are straddling your thigh. Gently bob partner up in the air by lifting yourself up and down with your right leg. Let go of the right wrist. As the unwrapping starts turn partner in a great circle with your hand under the head. While turning, switch hands under the head and come out on the right side, your right hand under the sacrum (Free Float). Hold perfectly still so that partner can experience stillness.

Additional Wallwork

1. Back Stretches

If you have a wall to lean back against, you can, in the middle of the session, back up against it while the person is in the Free Float position to work with your knee. This should not be done with anyone who has lower back problems. Hold the chest with your left hand, your left arm under the neck, and the far thigh with your right hand, your arm under the near leg. Work gently down the back with your right knee (your right foot braced on your left leg). Place your right knee against the left buttock and, letting partner lie on the left side, simultaneously pull the chest and thigh, being careful to not overextend the spine. When you remove the knee and partner is facing upward again, place your knee at the top of the leg and pull the leg down. Float out to bring around the other side, or do the Twist from Behind.

2.⊗ Twist from Behind

If the foot can be pushed down without hitting the bottom, when the leg is still pulled down, remove your knee from underneath and push the leg down between your legs. Clasp it between your thighs and hold the chest with your left hand while your right hand slowly rotates the right leg holding the thigh near the back of the knee. Rotate it across the front. Catch it in your left hand which pulls the right knee across while your right hand pulls the right shoulder back, to twist-stretch the spine. Release the left leg, letting partner float up to your left, and do the Back Stretches and the twist from this side, after which you can return to position 1.

Sideways at the Wall

A simple way of working at the wall is this position which can come in the middle or at the end of a session. While holding someone's knees to the chest in the first position, back up to the wall and brace the bottom of your right foot on your extended left leg. Lower the backs of the knees over your raised right thigh. Keeping the back straight, hold and work the head and neck with both hands. Float partner out or, if this is at the end, lower the feet to the ground and lean partner back against the wall.

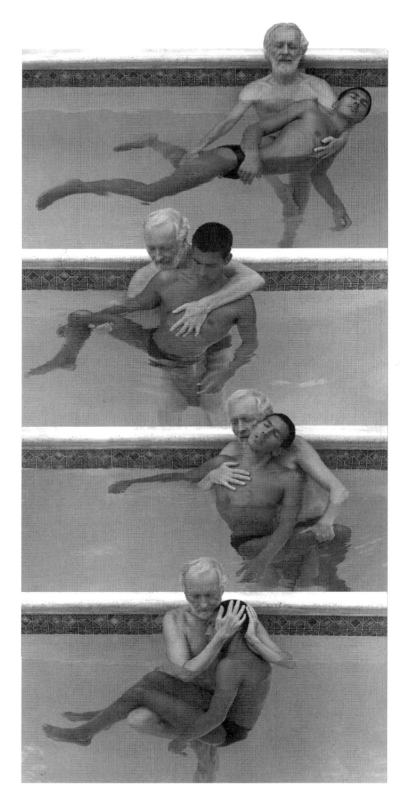

Stepwork

Ideally, steps have a wall alongside them that you can lean back against while sitting sideways on a step holding someone in front of you. If the steps are curved, it is best if they don't start curving until they are three feet out from the wall alongside. The following is a sequence that works very well on ideal steps. If you don't have a wall to lean back against, or steps that curve quickly, adapt this as best you can. Much of this sequence is similar to the sequence done from above the head when someone is on their side in Tantsu. I usually do it only on the one side described below, the side from which I can work with my right hand.

1. Sitting

If your pool has steps alongside a wall, back up to them holding your partner in position 1, the knees held close to the chest as in the accordion. Lean back against the wall to the right side of the steps. Leave room for the right arm between your lower back and the wall. Holding the knees as close to the chest as possible, clasp the back and thighs between your two legs. Hold. Pull your right arm out from under the knees and grab the far leg before it straightens out. Hold it to the chest and let the other leg straighten. Place your right foot on the step below, over and to the inside of the near leg. Let go of the other leg. Partner is comfortably straddling your lower calf, head resting against the upper left corner of your chest.

2. Face and Head

Holding under the occiput with your left hand, work freestyle around the face and over the skull with the four fingers of your right hand.

3. Neck and Shoulders

Squeeze down the neck. Work around the shoulder and under the shoulder blade, holding partner close to you the whole time.

4. Chest Opening

With your left hand pull the left shoulder back. If possible, hook the left elbow over your left knee behind partner. Work across the chest between the ribs with your four fingers.

5. Upper Back

Place your right hand on the heart center. Release the left arm and work down the bladder meridian in the upper back with your left thumb while holding the heart center with your right.

6. Shoulder Rotation

Clasp the left shoulder between the heels of your hands and slowly rotate.

7. Arm Rotation

Brace behind the left shoulder with the heel of your left hand, while you raise and rotate the left arm with your right hand. Lay the arm up over the head.

8. Side Opening

If the left arm stays over the head, stretching the left side open, you can work down that side and into the lower back, pulling with both hands together.

9.⊗ Leg Work

If you can reach and pull up the left leg, you can hold the ankle with your left hand and rotate the foot with your right. Propping it over your right leg, work up spleen meridian in the calf.

10. The Hara

Lay the neck back over your left knee and support the tailbone on your right knee. Squeeze and rock the lower back with your left hand while holding the hara with your right. Lay your left arm over the chest. Squeeze and work the hara with both hands.

11. On Both Knees

Staying on the steps, slip the arm out from behind your back and lie back holding the head in both hands, your two knees gently raised under the lower back. While rocking partner, stretched out over your knees, pull and turn the head and work the neck.

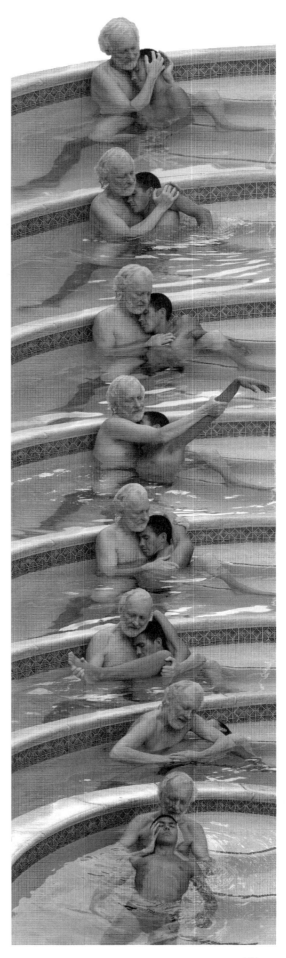

The Gyroscope

The Gyroscope is a move in which slowly turning, we lift someone out of the water and let them free fall back a moment. Don't do this with anyone who might get seasick or is too large for you to lift out. I often do this at the end of the Near Leg Over. Tugging the near thigh to slip the leg off your shoulder can lead into this move.

1.⊗ Gyroscope

Begin in position 1, your right arm over the top of the near thigh. Keep the thigh firmly clasped to your side, your right hand under the near hip as you start to slowly turn counter-clockwise. As you turn, lower your right side into the water, simultaneously lifting the torso into a vertical position. When partner is most vertical, raise your body while still turning to give the experience of momentarily free falling back into the water. Have your left hand ready to catch the head before the neck snaps back. Do not stop this slow turning until there are three or four free falls. After the last fall, hold partner across your chest. Stretch the spine by hooking the fingers of your right hand in the top of the sacrum and pulling while holding the occiput with your left forearm. Lay partner back in the water and do the Sacrum Rock.

2.⊗ Sacrum Rock

Do only with those with whom your arm is long enough to reach between their legs to the sacrum without pressing against their genitals. In position 1, while partner is floating on the back, hook your fingertips in the top of the sacrum.. Keeping the occiput firmly held in the crook of your elbow, rock partner head to toe, stretching the spine. Return to the Basic Moves.

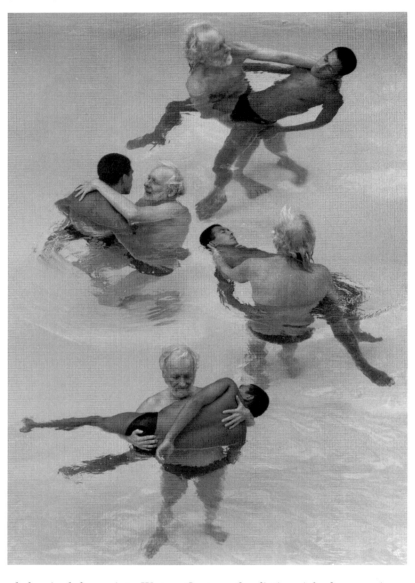

A Dancer's Watsu

Alexander Georgeakopoulos brings the grace of classical dance into Watsu. On top of a distinguished career in ballet, he studied Trager work and then, Watsu. What follows are notes he prepared for his students here at Harbin:

Lightness	Perceive and communicate through softness and gentleness that the body is weightless and can float lightly and freely. This is one of the greatest potentials of working in water.
Stillness in Movement, Movement in Stillness	Understand how the tempo at which one watsus fosters different reactions. Slower tempos relax and create awareness, giving time to feel, and do not distract one back from trance to the purely physical. Quicker tempos tend to stimulate and move energy. The question is how slowly can this form be watsued and still be in a movement flow? In moments of cradling, of rest, allow the movement to continue subtly as a reassuring continuity and presence.
Without agenda	Rather than beginning a Watsu, let the Watsu begin itself out of the experience of unity, what Milton Trager terms 'hook up' and describes as a connection with The All and the person one is with. Watsuing without agenda, there is no judgment, no need to accomplish anything. Limits and holding patterns can be accepted--one can play with them and see if they want to shift. Create a space into which a person can flow, to occupy as he/she wishes.

One movement   From beginning to end a Watsu is a single unbroken movement, ongoing, modulating, sometimes subtle, sometimes full and manifesting. This brings poetry, music and dance into the Watsu and the person feels him/herself as music, as if she were 'danced' or flying.

Roundedness   The body responds to curved, circular movements which are cyclic and unending vs. linear movements with a beginning and an end. Categorizing my moves, there are four types, which combine in practice, but can be broken down for purposes of understanding as follows:

Rainbows Half-circles on the horizontal plane, in which you rotate on your standing axis like a bullfighter and the watsuee moves around you

Pendulum swings The watsuee swings away from you and toward you, coming to a moment of stillness at the high point, accelerating into the trough, slowing down on the upswing; this rocking can be done with great sensitivity

Spirals On the horizontal plane, the watsuee is arched along the circumference of a circle

Waves Combining the horizontal and vertical planes, the watsuee is translated into a repeating wave pattern.

Polarities   **Arching vs. Rounding** As in yoga, arching movements to the spine are balanced by rounded movements. Time spent in moves in which the lower back is unsupported and hyperextended need to be followed by comforting, rounded holds.

Movement vs. Stillness Following active periods of movement in which the body is stretched and worked are rest periods of stillness during which assimilation takes place.

Close and held vs. Free and floating A profound lesson Watsu has to offer is that the safety and security of being cradled, held, and nurtured is equally available while floating free and unattached. An integration of the poles occurs which has to do with stepping out into life free of dependency, allowing nurturing in one's life, knowing there are no strings attached.

The Vortex

The Vortex is an example of what Alexander calls a spiral. Begin from above your partner's head. As you pull the right arm up above the head with your right hand, move to the left side of the head. Hold the occiput between the thumb and forefinger of your left hand, its palm turned upward, its thumb facing you. As one hand is pulling the arm, lift with the other forearm (your hand still holding the occiput) up under the upper back between the scapula and the spine so that there is a roll away from you, towards the arm you are pulling. As you let go of that arm, take up the other arm and roll the person from the other side of the head. Continue alternating, rolling from side to side. As with Alexander's other moves there is a precision of footwork and stance, an awareness of how one's own spine is held and interacting, which have their origin in classical dance. Their is a lifting, an aerial quality which adds a counterpoint to Watsu's basic sinking and surrendering into the water.

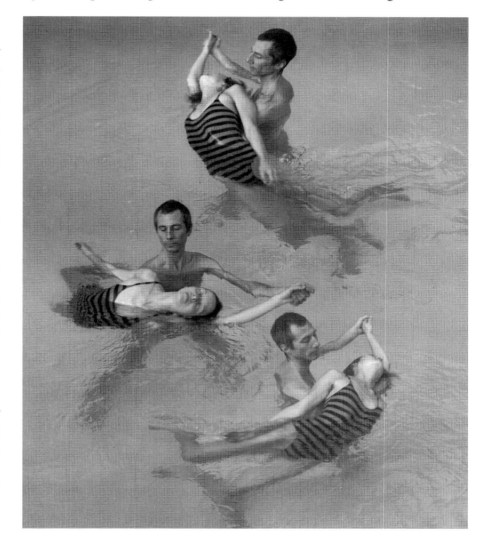

Elaine Marie

Elaine Marie's power as watsuer and teacher comes through Alma Flor Ada's account of sessions and classes with her in Chapter VIII. Having to work in a pool that is deep for her, and often with people larger than her, she has developed many moves, such as the following, which are neither size nor depth graded.

Seaweed

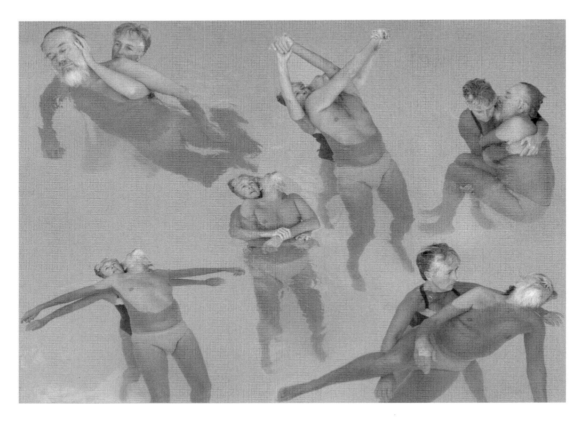

Begin under the head, holding it in both hands. Pull the body through the water like seaweed. Cross the arms and lift up. The arms still crossed, place the hands on the sides of the body. Bring the knees up and hold partner close to you, folded and protected in your arms. Keeping one arm under the occiput and the other under the near leg, slowly roll partner out to lie as still, and as lightly supported, as possible, released into the universe.

FREE FLOW

Rhythm of the energy being released

Finding the body, following, not leading, following whatever flow it leads us into, dancing to the rhythm of the energy being released, is freeing the body. The more we are centered in our own body and are one with the movement that flows out of that center, the more we can hold someone in our arms and be with the freedom in both our bodies. It is a very tangible, very loving freedom.

Surrendering

Surrendering to this freedom is the basis of Free Flow. The more you find a continuous, uninterrupted flow leading you through the Transition Flow, the easier it will be for you to let that same kind of flow lead you through ever new positions, slowly moving and stretching the body against and around yours in ever new ways. Don't force it. If you try to make it happen it is not free. You can be freer holding a point perfectly still than when trying to make Free Flow happen. Free Flow happens. It is always happening. Our bodies are like the most basic units of matter, simultaneously particle and wave. Our everyday perception of our bodies is as particles. In Free Flow we move to the body's wave. If this has not already begun to happen in our Transition Flow, we will not be able to move into Free Flow outside a sequence. When it does begin to happen there will be a like freedom in all of our Watsu.

Without intention

When you feel Free Flow carry you outside of sequence, let it, but feel free to be led back into sequence at any time. Don't let your ego trap you into feeling you have to prove how inventive and creative you can always be. Intention can only get in the way. Stay empty. That emptiness or void, and the creativity that rises out of it, are as much two aspects of the same thing as particle and wave.

CHAPTER VII

THE REHABILITATIVE BENEFITS OF WATSU

by Lisa Dougherty, Emily Dunlap and Sunny Mehler

This chapter is written by three authors who view Watsu in a western perspective: Lisa who discusses the effects that the elements in a Watsu have on the neurologically involved client; Emily, who addresses how the mind and body are connected and the ways in which Watsu effects both in order to allow for holistic healing; Sunny, who will share the importance of the unconditional stroking* and acceptance that is experienced in a Watsu and the implications that has for healing. Each of us brings our own perspective in our assessment of Watsu. These assessments are based on our own personal and professional life experiences. At this point, we will introduce ourselves in order to offer a better insight on how we view the importance of Watsu as a supplemental form of treatment. Then we will present case studies followed by our individual comments.

Lisa Dougherty

Hello, my name is Lisa Dougherty. I was born and raised in a small mid-western town (Leavenworth, Kansas), the fifth of six children of a close-knit Catholic family. I earned a Bachelors degree in Human Biology at the University of Kansas, and a Masters degree in Physical Therapy at the Kansas University Medical Center. Upon completion of my physical therapy degree I came to Timpany Center (a private, non-profit aquatic therapy facility in San Jose, California) to begin my career as a therapist.

Experiencing Watsu

It was at Timpany that I viewed a Watsu for the first time. I must admit that my conservative upbringing left me feeling a little shocked and embarrassed by the physical closeness required to perform the Watsu. My "Western - Put it in writing and prove it" education made me leery of the medical benefits this "Eastern - Woo Woo" technique could possess. Upon receiving a Watsu I had a complete paradigm shift. I no longer was embarrassed by the physical closeness that I had misinterpreted from afar, but welcomed the very nurturing arms that cradled me like a baby as I was floated through the water on one of the most relaxing journeys I had ever experienced. Soon my 'Western' educated mind realized that the nature of the Watsu moves performed in the water were very similar to the basis of Physical Therapy techniques used with neurologically involved clients.

Watsu's effect on the primary sensory systems

The stretching and rotation movements of the trunk and limbs, along with the effects of the water rushing in and out of the ears, lights playing on the eyelids as the head rolls from side to side, and temperature changes on the skin from warm water to the cooler air circulating above; effect the same primary sensory systems (kinesthetic, proprioceptive, vestibular and tactile) used in popular Physical Therapy techniques like NDT (Neurologic Developmental Technique), Rood and PNF (Proprioceptive Neuromuscular Facilitation). The above mentioned sensory systems effected by Watsu and the Physical Therapy techniques are used to facilitate* active/normal motor responses; and it was because of this similar connection that I incorporate the Watsu into the hydrotherapy treatment of the neurologically involved.

* Terms followed by an asterisk are defined in the glossary at the end of this chapter.

Emily Dunlap

Hello, my name is Emily Dunlap. I was born and raised in Boston, Massachusetts, where I earned my Physical Therapy degree at Simmons College. My early work experience had been in a rehabilitational hospital where I treated a variety of people with differing diagnoses, such as: geriatric orthopedic (arthritis, joint replacements); neorologic (spinal cord injury, head trauma, strokes); and chronic pain. I performed therapy treatments both in and out of the water. I am extremely impressed by the positive effects that aquatic treatment has for my clients. I feel that the therapeutic benefits of water, combined with quality treatment, is a powerful facilitator of well being. This is why I sought out Timpany Center.

Empowering the client

In my experience as a PT, I have noticed that recovery from a physical illness or injury is greatly influenced by a person's psychological or emotional state. I have seen over and over again where people who have positive attitudes show a quicker recovery than someone with a negative outlook or unresolved emotional traumas. I also feel that an important part of my treatment is just being close to a person, showing them that you care and using a hands-on approach to facilitate a positive change both physically and psychologically. This, in conjunction with proper education, will empower the client and encourage a lifelong change toward well being.

For me, Watsu is a wonderful treatment which encourages both physical and psychological healing. As we go over the case studies I will give my impressions of why Watsu is so powerful.

Sunny Mehler

Hello, my name is Sunny Mehler. I was born and raised in Birmingham, Alabama. My interest in Eastern thinking first began in my studies at the University of Alabama, where I earned my Bachelor's Degree. My interest in eastern philosophy was rediscovered through associations made during my training in Transactional Analysis at Grouphouse, Inc., Western Institute of Psychotherapy for Families and Groups, and membership in the International Transactional Analysis Association. For 18 years, I have been facilitating groups using the concepts in Corrective Parenting, a form of Transactional Analysis. During this time, whether I was counseling families in a crises intervention setting, facilitating individuals in a group setting, or teaching students in a classroom setting--one very basic element continued to be of paramount importance: the element of unconditional 'ok'ness.' The opportunity to experience this quality is that which creates my enthusiasm for Watsu. People who are dealing with chronic pain sometimes find that their conditions are deeply rooted in unresolved emotional issues. Others are dealing with 'normal everyday stress'. The beauty of Watsu is, regardless of what the case may be, the prescription reads: "May be given as needed."

The western paradigm

The most difficult aspect in discussing Watsu within the realm of Western medicine is that Watsu is a holistic and Eastern form of healing. Part of the difficulty arises in that holistic thinking and practices have previously been foreign to the western mind. The western paradigm is to specialize; to separate mind, body and spirit in order to examine them in finer detail. This is demonstrated by our specialized disciplines in Medicine, Psychology and Religion. An advantage to this kind of specialization has been acquiring a knowledge base that has proven valuable in dealing with acute traumas or in identifying and in some instances eliminating diseases. Though modern science continues to advance and make astonishing discoveries in these specialized areas, there are times when a condition will not heal, but rather becomes chronic. Whether it is the mind influencing the body, or the body influencing the mind is unclear; however, it is clear that combining the knowledge base from various disciplines makes the healing process more complete and satisfactory. It is with this thinking and consciousness that Watsu be considered as a supplementary method to be used in conjunction with the present medical treatments and psychological interventions being employed.

In Watsu, because it is multi-dimensional, the participants have the opportunity for addressing their physical, psychological and spiritual needs to the degree that they will allow. As Harold stated earlier, all of us are influenced by our paradigms and so our experiences vary. A Watsu experience can be a subtle form of healing, or it can be a most profound and consciousness-raising experience. It influences and uniquely blends both the physical and the psychological needs of the recipient. What continues to be of prime importance is that, regardless of the initial paradigm that a person may have, most participants feel nourished by this experience.

*Timpany
Center
clientele*

At Timpany Center, we see many people who are suffering from aches and pains of the body and/or mind. Our clientele varies greatly, from young children with learning disabilities to older adults with chronic pain. For these clients, Watsu has been used either alone, or in conjunction with Physical Therapy treatments with great success. We have chosen the following case studies to demonstrate the wide spectrum to which Watsu is applicable. The clients names have been changed to protect their confidentiality.

Case Study 1 - Joe

History

Joe is a 32 year old male, who suffered a closed head injury (brain stem); and left arm dislocation and/or fracture in an auto accident two years prior to initial evaluation at Timpany Center. Joe has severe muscle contractures* of left arm and hand, minimum to moderate contractures of right arm, and moderate to severe contractures of inner thigh muscles due to increased muscle tone* as a side effect of his brain injury. His legs and feet have excessive extensor* tone (increased when angry or excited), and the arms are held curled in close to the chest. Joe appears to understand most of what is said to him, but is often inappropriate with his response. He presently is in the abusive stage (verbally and physically) of his head injury. Accurate strength and range* of motion measurements were not taken upon evaluation due to increased tone and contractures of arms and legs, as well as Joe's willingness/ability to understand commands. At home, Joe is performing stretching exercises (with his wife), and is in a standing frame for an hour a day. He is in a wheelchair and is dependent for most daily activities.

*Treatment after
injury*

Prior to Aquatic Physical Therapy treatment, Joe had received two years of physical therapy rehabilitation on land without any significant gains to recovery. Joe's family reported they believe this was largely due to the excessive amounts of tone and contractures, as well as Joe's abusive (physical and verbal) behavior.

*Aquatic
Physical
Therapy*

Joe's hydrotherapy treatment sessions initially consisted of weight-bearing exercises in a 'water walker' (flotation device) and passive ranging of arms and active/assistive of legs. With these exercises, client often resisted stretching of limbs, and had many abusive outbursts.

Watsu Therapy

After approximately three weeks of treatment sessions of this kind, the Watsu technique was incorporated into the program. Because of Joe's excessive amounts of tone and contractures, only the initial movements of the first stage of Watsu could be performed; but the gentle rotation of the trunk through the water while ranging the legs into flexion* and extension* had a dramatic effect on decreasing the tone in the legs. It was also noted that the Watsu had a very calming effect on Joe's behavior, and he became more cooperative with attempting to perform the exercises. In approximately four months time of combined treatments of Watsu and traditional hydrotherapy exercises Joe was able to perform; alternate hip and knee flexion/extension independently while supine; pull to standing in water walker with minimum to moderate assistance at hips and knees; and the incident of abusive outburst had decreased dramatically. At this time the client began physical therapy treatment on land to continue to improve trunk stability and weight bearing tolerance.

*Wife's
comments*

Joe's wife commented, "Joe came to Timpany Center and was pretty stiff and having a lot of cramps. Joe's therapist decided to try the Watsu program hoping it would help ease his cramps and loosen the muscles so he could get more movement with less pain, which was keeping Joe from improving his condition. Since Joe's experience with this program I feel he was able to manage less pain and has a lot more movement in his legs. I feel it's worth trying this program. Joe is on his way back to a better life with more movement and less pain."

Comments (Lisa)

Effects on muscle tone

The effects of Watsu on the sensory system played a large part in reducing the tone of the trunk and legs of Joe. The sensory input of touch in a Watsu can be used to facilitate or inhibit* desired or undesired responses through the receptors located in the skin, muscles, tendons, joints and inner ears by relaying information about movement to the reticular activating system which determines a person's level of response. A slow, rhythmical rocking/rolling movement applied using firm but light constant contact, in general will have an inhibiting effect on increased muscle tone. An abrupt, repetitive movement involving quick stretches has a tendency to facilitate or enhance muscle tone.

Neurological treatment techniques

Inhibiting abnormal tone for increased range of motion/mobility, and facilitating stability, posture, and normal movement patterns are major treatment goals of neurological treatment techniques such as PNF, Rood and NDT. The rhythmic rotation of head (inner ear), trunk, and limbs with Watsu promotes integration of tonic reflexes* and stimulates the righting reactions (balance) needed to maintain posture with sitting, and eventually standing.

Traction and approximation

In Watsu, when the arms and legs are passively stretched, * forces are applied to the joints. Traction at the joint promotes mobility and flexion of the surrounding muscles; and approximation of the joint reinforces stability and extension of the surrounding muscles. This passive stimulation to the joints applied in Watsu sets up the groundwork for the muscles surrounding the joint to perform actively. Eventually it is the combination of mobility/stability and the active co-contraction of flexion/extension of the muscles that allows a person to advance to the level of performing normal movement patterns or skills.

Watsu's most significant benefit

In closing, I would like to comment that incorporating the Watsu technique in the treatment program of the neurologically involved client will promote increased range of motion by breaking up excessive flexor* and/or extensor patterns, and initiate the beginning stages of developing righting reactions and trunk stability; but the most significant benefit I feel Watsu has to offer is the nurturing, unconditional acceptance experienced with a Watsu that allows a person to let go of some of the frustrations of the mind and emotional state, which in turn can have a profound effect on that person's attitude and their approach to life.

Case Study 2 - Jane

History

52 year old woman who was referred to Timpany Center with a diagnosis of fibromyalgia* and degenerative disc disease in her neck. Her past medical history included low back pain and lumbar* surgery (lumbar fusion*). Jane reported having a history of depression and had seen a psychiatrist in the past. She had a sleeping disorder for more than two years and required medication to get a full night's sleep. Due to depression, work stress (caused by difficulty interacting with her supervisor), and complaints of pain in her hips and upper back, she has been off of work for three months.

Watsu and aquatic exercise

For one month Watsu treatments were administered once a week in addition to water exercise in class setting. She reported a noticeable improvement with her sleeping pattern and was able to get a full night sleep without taking medication.

Aquatic physical therapy and Watsu

At this point, an evaluation was given by a physical therapist. The evaluation showed moderate limitations of the flexibility in her back and neck, as well as moderate tightness in her legs and arms. Jane reported that her tightness had improved since starting Watsu and water exercise, but it was still a problem. She was deconditioned and had severe weakness in her back and hips. Jane held much tension in her upper back, of which she was unaware. When asked to relax she would release her shoulders, but as soon as she was distracted, the tension would come back. She reported being able to walk only 10-30 minutes before the pain would increase.

84

At this point, Jane initiated aquatic physical therapy twice a week and continued with the Watsu treatments once a week.

Work stress

In two months, Jane noted a dramatic decrease in her level of pain. She reported being able to walk three hours at a time with no increase of pain, and was able to sleep through the night without medication. She had improved flexibility and strength in her hips, back and neck. Her endurance improved as well. At this point she returned to work full time. Unfortunately, her pain symptoms gradually started to return and she reported that she unconsciously clenched her fist throughout the night and woke up each morning with severe wrist pain (carpal tunnel syndrome). She was still having difficulties interacting with her supervisor and realized that her pain symptoms were directly related to work stress. Presently she has been participating in independent aquatic exercise to maintain her strength and endurance and reports that Watsu helps to reduce her anxiety, increase her flexibility, and improve her sleeping pattern.

Case Study 3 - Mary

History

62 year old female came to Timpany Center with a one year old rotator cuff* injury and muscle spasms in her right shoulder. She had injured her right shoulder in the Northern California earthquake in 1989.

Treatment after injury

Mary received traditional Physical Therapy for 2-3 treatments, consisting of ultrasound* and gentle exercises. This treatment was discontinued because her pain increased and she showed decreased range of motion in her right shoulder.

Aquatic Physical Therapy

Mary came to Timpany Center two to three times a week for 3 months. Treatments included supervised and independent active water exercise with emphasis on stretching, strengthening and massage therapy. After this treatment improvements were noted with pain and increased flexibility in her right shoulder (see chart below). However, she continued with significant pain and tightness in her shoulder which interfered with her daily activities and quality of life. At this point, she was referred to receive Watsu treatments.

Watsu Therapy

After having 5 Watsu treatments, Mary showed a dramatic increase in the flexibility of her right shoulder (see chart below), decreased pain and muscle guarding, improved posture and breathing pattern.

The following chart provides goiniometric measurements taken of the right shoulder at different times during her treatment

Right Shoulder ROM	9-5-90	10-10-90	11-13-90	12-12-90
	initial PT eval	PT re-eval	PT re-eval	after 5 Watsus
flexion	0-90	0-110	0-105	0-150
abduction	0-85	0-100	0-80	0-135
external rotation	0-30	0-60	0-45	0-65
internal rotation	0-30	0-30	0-65	not measured

Mary's impressions of her Watsu treatments

After the first Watsu

"It is one thing to watch Watsu, quite another to experience it. From the outside it seems rather weird, a body being manipulated in the water, yet there is something beautiful, too. The movements are so fluid. My first impression was of closeness to the guide. The intimacy seems greater than that of being massaged, perhaps it is because you are both in swimsuits, both in the water. You are very close to another person and that person takes you and holds you as a mother might. After I got over a certain awkwardness at the intimacy, I was overcome by the back to the womb experience. This, I thought, was how it might have been before I was born. Totally taken care of, nothing to worry about, nothing to do anything about except go with the flow. This is difficult for one used to being in control, to give up that control. It took most of the first session to learn how to do that."

"I came to this Watsu 'experienced', knowing what to expect; but I soon found out the Watsu experience is never quite the same. True, I found it easier to let go and much more pleasant. The more I let go, the more things floated to the surface of my mind. I might have been taking mental therapy, for things from my childhood surfaced, some pleasant, some not so pleasant, but I felt while my body was in limbo. I was learning about myself. I wanted it to go on forever. I wanted to bottle it up and take it home with me. I was very relaxed, especially for the tense person that I usually am. I felt calm and in control."

"I came to the third session in a great deal of pain. I wasn't sure how it would go since the pain had kept me awake most of the night. I was, therefore, on guard. At first I was only aware of the pain in my right arm and my desire to protect it from anything that might cause further pain. This made it more difficult to let go. But, frankly, the movements are so beautiful, especially for one like me who has never been able to dance, that eventually the fluidity of my body in the water and the arms I was in, felt so safe and secure, they lulled me into submission. Approximately two-thirds through the session I realized that the pain was gone. I felt like laughing out loud, but I didn't for fear of breaking the spell."

Comments (Emily)

Emotions have a profound effect on the body's tissues and can aid in their facilitating or impeding recovery. To demonstrate this, I will discuss Case Study #2. Jane reported that she had been under a great deal of stress at work because she had difficulty interacting with her supervisor. Work and everyday stresses had become so intense that she took a leave of absence from work and began counseling with a psychiatrist who diagnosed her with having clinical depression. The stress that Jane experienced was effecting her body in many ways. The most noticeable physiological change was muscle tension or prolonged muscle contraction in her upper trapezius muscles (shoulder). Normally the body is an excellent self healing machine which is in a constant state of dynamic homeostasis. But if a continuous stress is placed on the body over a prolonged period of time the body's tissues will change to accommodate this stress. In Jane's case the prolonged muscle tension in her trapezius* muscle eventually changed the physiologic make-up of the muscle, distorting the balance of chemicals in the muscle, changing the composition of cell types (fast twitch vs. slow twitch), changing the vascular structures of the muscles, etc., thereby changing the biomechanics of the muscle. This will also effect the surrounding tissues. The nerves traveling nearby the muscle were compressed by the constant muscle contraction, possibly causing pain. Nearby blood vessels were also compressed, thereby effecting the blood supply going to and from the muscle. Connective tissue adaptively shortened and distorted, while conforming to the prolonged changes from the increased muscle tension. The prolonged muscle tension effected the bony structure of the neck by causing compression of the cervical spine which aggravated and possibly facilitated the degenerative disc disease in Jane.

Pain caused by the degenerative disc disease started another type of cycle which was difficult for Jane to break. When in pain, a person often becomes immobile to prevent increasing the pain. She avoided daily activities which involved lifting, prolonged sitting, standing or repetitive movements. With this inactivity came muscle tightness and weakness. Jane had difficulty doing the activities that she used to do easily, i.e., grocery shopping, going out to dinner with friends, working. This led to psycho/social/economical problems, such as decreased self-esteem because she could no longer function in her job, decreased interaction with her friends and family because she felt that they were tired of hearing her complain, and was not able to participate in social activities due to physical limitations. This isolated Jane from others and led to deeper depression. She also suffered from stress caused by economical issues, such as less income while on leave of absence, medical bills which needed to be paid, frustrations with medical insurance and workmen's compensation, etc. These added to the stress that Jane was presently under and translated into more muscle tension.

Below is a diagram of a pain cycle showing how physical, social, economical and psychological dysfunctions effect each other.

PSYCHO/SOCIAL/ECONOMICAL   PHYSICAL

Stress → Muscle Tension → Pain → Immobility → Weakness → Tightness → Decreased functional activities → Financial difficulties → Isolation/depression → Low self esteem → Stress

Embarassment and depression

This cycle is just one example of how the body and mind interact. Another example would be a physically disabled client who is embarrassed because he is no longer 'normal'. His embarrassment causes him to avoid eye contact with other people effecting this posture and isolating him from others. Another example would be someone who is depressed and uses food to satisfy their need for pleasure. This person may end up with a significant weight problem which impacts upon their physical wellness.

Breaking the cycles

Watsu provides a channel to break into these cycles of physical/psychological dysfunctions. The nurturing aspects of Watsu often have a dramatic effect on that person's self-esteem and sense of OK'ness. This may be enough to allow the client to release muscle tension that they were holding, which was the experience that Mary (case study #3) discussed when giving her impressions of Watsu.

Stored emotions

Some people feel that emotions of traumatic events can be stored in the body's tissues. The extensive stretching and slow rhythmical movements in Watsu aids in the release of tissue distortion which can cause the surfacing of these emotions. Once surfaced, these emotions can be acknowledged and possibly resolved. A good example of this would be the memory of sexual abuse held in the body's tissues as tension or distortion which keeps the trunk flexed and the arms and legs held in close to the body. This person carries the tension/distortion without realizing. They assume this posture in an attempt to keep their body closed, not allowing others to invade their privacy. In a Watsu session, this person may experience difficulty with the wide open movements, until they let go. Once allowing the tissues to release they may experience reliving or remembering the sexual abuse. When realizing they can remember the abuse without falling apart, knowing that they are OK, they are able to release the tension which had been holding them in a closed posture.

Benefits of warm water

Warm water has many therapeutic benefits. Superficial circulation increases in warm water; this will decrease pain and increase the pliability of soft tissues, allowing for greater range of motion with stretching. The buoyancy of the water unloads the joints, often lessening pain, allowing for greater flexibility. Water in the ears muffles auditory distractions from the outer environment, allowing for greater relaxation and body awareness.

Relaxation and breath

In Watsu, with the ears under the water . . . eyes closed . . . body flowing smoothly from one move to the other, the client becomes aware of the level of relaxation they can attain. This relaxation will enhance their breathing pattern, allowing for slow, rhythmical, deep breaths, rather than short, quick, shallow breaths which often accompany stress. During the Watsu session the client has time to learn about themselves, without any distraction, demands or needs from the outside world.

Case Study 4 - Joe

History

Joe is a 40 year old male, presently in his second marriage and the father of a 20-year-old daughter. He is the oldest of seven boys and comes from a very dysfunctional and alcoholic home, with physical, emotional, verbal and sexual abuse. Joe is also a recovering alcoholic/addict with almost six years of sobriety training through 12-Step programs and five years of private therapy. He is currently working in a chemical dependency hospital as an addiction counselor. Joe has chronic back pain and had been seen at Timpany Center for aquatic physical therapy and Watsu treatments.

Impressions after Watsu

"My first two Watsu sessions were very relaxing and soothing, but my level of trust was low and I wasn't able to totally surrender and get the most out of them. About six weeks ago, I started getting in touch with some very painful memories and feelings from my childhood and I wanted to access more of the emotional component, so I set up extra psychotherapy sessions and body work, including massage and Watsu. I went into my Watsu session with a willingness to surrender to whatever came up.

Abandonment pain

"In one Watsu session following a very traumatic therapy session using regressive guided memory, I was able to be in touch with a great amount of abandonment pain as my Watsu practitioner was cradling me. I was able to cry and let the pain go and felt a sense of release. As the session ended I felt very young and totally relaxed and was in touch with a sense of well being. In another session, I was able to get in touch with some rather pleasant childhood memories that had been blocked out. I plan to continue to use Watsu to help me unlock and to be in touch with memories and emotions that are difficult for me to access with psychotherapy alone."

Comments (Sunny)

Watsu provides an experience of 'unconditional acceptance' which can encourage individuals to seek this kind of attention in other areas of their life. Even though the above client was seen in physical therapy, his impression speaks to the psychological benefits that he experienced.

Unconditional acceptance

In exploring the value of Watsu as a supplemental treatment, patients have been asked to record their impressions and the results of their Watsu experiences. In almost every case, the results were positive. The most consistently acknowledged aspects in the treatments were intimacy and 'unconditional acceptance'. This is not surprising, because from the day that we are born, this is a fundamental physical and psychological need. After food, physical closeness and nurturing is the next most vital element in good health and survival for the infant. Yet many of the clients interviewed openly admitted that they were not accustomed to 'unconditional acceptance'. That their sense of OK'ness came from their ability to do, how well they perform, or how good they look. That, in fact, their OK'ness from their perspective is conditional. The implication is that the world is full of people trying to figure out how to be loved and accepted. There are many who think they have figured it out within their family system or their circle of friends. They perform accordingly but then something happens. They get hurt or fall ill and can no longer perform in those ways that gave them the recognition that they were earning. For many, being sick or hurt is the only way they have permission to allow themselves to be cared for by others. Through psychological treatment, these perceptions, and the problems that result from them, can be changed or resolved. For some of these people, Watsu nourishes this need for physical, unconditional and positive stroking. In their Watsu experience, the nonverbal message is that this need is OK and natural. As a result of this permission, they find that they are enabled to pursue this kind of unconditional recognition and acceptance in other areas of their lives. There are few ways in our society in which people can share an intimate and nourishing exchange with another person without a list of conditions that have to be met in order to make that kind of interaction socially acceptable or safe. Watsu offers that kind of opportunity to people who literally do not know one another; yet with 'no strings attached'. This kind of 'unconditional acceptance' can lead to authenticity and the expression of the true self. It is kind of 'openness' that often leads to health and is the quality that people would like to share with their families.

Though society is heavily weighted in rewarding 'doing', there exists a need in people for the unconditional acceptance of who they are just for their being. Those families who are receiving counseling for the many problems that plague families today can find the use of Watsu as a nice supplement to other therapies being employed.

Watsu and family therapy

Recovering from sexual abuse

Using the structure of Watsu among family members would offer them a way to learn to be close with 'no strings attached'. This can be a supplemental form of healing used in conjunction with psychotherapy for those families who are recovering from sexual abuse. Anyone who lives with injunctions of "Don't be close" (because it's not safe) can experience a closeness in Watsu that is nurturing to offset previous experiences that have been painful. Many people only know 'being close' through a sexual experience; Watsu offers a way of being close without being sexual.

OK'ness

Often we hear people seeking a respite where they can 'just be themselves'. Imagine a world where people can experience just being themselves. That their 'being' is OK just because they 'are'. That a distinction is made between behavior and the person. That a behavior being exhibited may need to change, but that a person's OK'ness is never in question. That thought is very healing.

Though society rewards doing (families, friends and even yourself) what most people hunger for is the 'unconditional acceptance' of who they are just for their being. If people have learned to believe that they are only conditionally OK; that they have to earn the strokes they need and now they can no longer perform; how will this affect their stroke supply and their sense of OK'ness? It seems that it will diminish their self-esteem.

Parent/Infant Watsu

In recognizing the importance of unconditional stroking and acceptance, a Parent/Infant Watsu class is offered at Timpany Center for families with disabled infants. Most of the parents involved are trained by their attending therapists in administering different exercises or techniques to their babies for the particular disability that they have. One of the prerequisites for this class is that the parents receive a Watsu first. In receiving the Watsu first, the parent then understands that this is an experience they are sharing with their child rather than a technique they're doing to their child. Watsu, for them, becomes an experience of bonding and intimacy with their babies in a healing but most spontaneous and even playful way. One of the most poignant moments in class was watching a young, powerfully-built father share a gentle Watsu with his 14 month old daughter who has cerebral palsy. They were completely focused on each other, like in a dance. This was an experience they were sharing; yet it offered all of the benefits of previously prescribed exercises that were usually done to the child.

Though Watsu's versatility offers multiple benefits to a variety of people, there are some contraindications for particular conditions. Some benefits and contraindications follow:

Benefits of Watsu	**Who can benefit from Watsu**
Decrease muscle guarding/tension	Acute/subacute/chronic pain
Increase range of motion	Neuromuscular disorders
Decrease pain	Head injury
Increase superficial circulation	Soft tissue dysfunction
Improve breathing pattern	Chronic headaches
Improve posture	Chronic fatigue
Normalize tone	Hyperactivity
Reduce stress/anxiety	Stress/anxiety related disorders
Improve body awareness	Depression
Discovery/release of emotional stress	Victims of mental, physical or sexual abuse
Improve sleeping pattern	Sleeping disorders
Increase energy/less fatigue	Substance abuse/addictions

Contraindications to Watsu

Absolute Contraindications - not appropriate for aquatic therapy
- fever over 100 degrees
- uncontrolled epilepsy
- cardiac failure
- significant open wounds
- respiratory disease of vital capacity less than 1500 cm2
- severe urinary tract infection
- severe respiratory tract infection
- blood infection
- tracheostomy
- bowel incontinence
- menstruation without internal protection
- infectious disease

Relative Contraindications - may not be appropriate / necessary precaution may need to be taken
- skin infections with drainage
- small open wounds (can be covered with tegrederm)
- uncontrolled blood pressure (moderate high blood pressure OK, but be careful with low blood pressure; ask doctor)
- unstable angina, cardiac arrythmias or additional cardiac considerations (ask doctor if it would be appropriate to go in warm water)
- intravenous lines, heplocks, hichman line, external collection devices (ask doctor)
- cerebral hemorrhage (should wait at least 3 weeks after bleeding has ceased; ask doctor)
- multiple sclerosis - may not tolerate warm water well (depends on client)
- chlorine sensitivity
- absence of cough reflex (would need to be monitored closely)
- dizziness (see below - vertigo)
- behavior problems - inappropriate physical, verbal or sexual behavior

Range of motion precautions - ask doctor if Watsu would be appropriate for client
- recent total hip replacement
- recent spinal surgery
- recent surgery
- acute ligamentous instability
- recent bone fracture
- arthritic cervical spine (be very careful with neck position, especially hyperextension)

Pain with spinal or peripheral joint range of motion - many can be treated with modifications to Watsu technique, just ask client to give feedback during the Watsu if a particular movement is aggravating their symptoms
- back/neck pain - bulged/herniated disc, facet irritation, spondylolethesis, arthritis (avoid extreme positions of spine)
- fibromyalgia
- frequent ear infections - may be appropriate to use ear plugs or medication

Excessive vertigo (dizziness) or other vestibular disorders - need to move slowly and monitor client's tolerance frequently, especially with first Watsu. To check tolerance, ask client to open eyes during Watsu and check for nystagmus (involuntary rhymical movement of the eyes back and forth), as well as asking if client feels dizzy or nauseous.

Inappropriate expression of Watsu - If client or practitioner feels uncomfortable with the physical closeness and intimacy of Watsu, or views Watsu as a sexual experience and acts inappropriately, may need to discuss the inappropriate behavior or discontinue Watsu.

Glossary

Approximation	the act or process of bringing closer together.
Carpal tunnel syndrome	condition involving inflammation, nerve compression, pain and muscle weakness in the wrist.
Contracture	a condition of fixed high resistance to passive stretch of a muscle, resulting from fibrosis of the tissues supporting the muscles or the joints, or from disorders of the muscle fibers.
Extension	a) the movement by which the two elements of any jointed part are drawn away from each other; b) a movement which brings the members of a limb into or toward a straight relation.
Extensor	a general term for any muscle that extends a joint (extensor pattern is when the surrounding muscles of several joints are involved).
Facilitation	the promotion or hastening of any natural process.
Fibromyalgia	a soft tissue disorder characterized by stiffness and joint or muscle pain, with swelling of the muscle tissues and the fiber-like connective tissues.
Flexion	the act of bending or condition of being bent.
Flexor	any muscle that flexes a joint (Flexor pattern is when the surrounding muscles of several joints are involved).
Inhibit	to retard, arrest or restrain.
Lumbar	referring to the part of the body between the chest and the pelvis, particularly the lower back area.
Lumbar fusion	surgery to the low back which involves fusing two or more lumbar vertebrae.
Range	the movement through which a joint can be extended and flexed.
Receptor	a sensory nerve terminal that responds to stimuli of various kinds.
Rotator cuff injury	injury to the tendons and muscles surrounding the shoulder joint.
Stroking	Strokes are units of recognition (physical, verbal, unconditional, conditional). That the need for them is universal is demonstrated by the dread of solitary confinement even the most hardened criminals feel. There are different levels of stroking: a) Self-stroking (daydreaming, meditating, withdrawal); b) Rituals; c) Pastiming; d) activities/work; e) psychological games; and f) intimacy.
Supine	lying face up.
Tone	the normal degree of vigor and tension; in muscle, the resistance to passive elongation or stretch. (Extensor tone - the muscles hold the joints in a straightened condition. Flexor tone - the muscles hold the joint in a bent position).
Tonic Reflexes	reflexes normally out-grown as toddlers, but often return with neurologically involved injuries.
Traction	the act of drawing or exerting a pulling force, as along the long axis of a structure.
Trapezius	a large, flat, triangular muscle of the shoulder and upper back. It raises the shoulder and flexes the arm.
Ultrasound	physical therapy treatment which utilizes sound waves to heat tissues and promote healing.

CHAPTER VIII

DANCING IN THE WATERS
a Woman's Watsu

by Alma Flor Ada

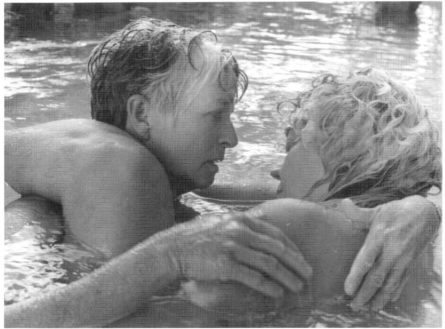

Miriam Grosman

To Elaine Marie
*Thank you for embracing me
in the love of the One Heart*

WATSU

The body, held in buoyancy
by gentle cradling arms returns
to lost memories of love without uncertainty.
The soul soars experiencing the freedom
of a body surrendered to the water--
in search of higher planes.
But it's not separation that occurs
rather, the extasis of Oneness.
Inside the floating body
the soul is free to sing
and the body
having defeated gravity
and all material ties
free from all bondage
returns to being essence
in your arms.

Spring has come early to Harbin this year. The early sun is uncovering hillsides purple with flowering lupine. I am anxious to get to the pools, yet I sit at the computer struggling to find words to describe experiences that transcend words. I feel honored and joyful to be part of this book and share my personal discoveries through Watsu.

At 52 years of age, I thought my life was at its zenith. I had achieved success as a full professor in a well-established university. I had many books published and received a number of honors. I had developed a rich connection with many of my students and graduates, who had become good friends, colleagues and co-authors. In addition I had established myself as a writer of fiction for children.

My family life also had a fullness, a like ripeness. My fourth child, my youngest son, had just graduated from college, as had his sister and two older brothers. But even more importantly, they had all bloomed to be responsible professionals and excellent human beings, compassionate, generous, self-sufficient and loving. With an unhappy first marriage well behind me, I was now married to a kind and understanding husband, a charming man.

One day my husband, Jorgen, proposed that before beginning the academic year, we take a few days to 'honeymoon' along the Mendocino coast. He arranged for us to start our vacation at Harbin Hot Springs, a resort community built around mineral springs that had been held sacred by Native American Indians. We had never been there, but my daughter, Rosalma, had spoken to us about Watsu, a form of massage done in the water at Harbin. When Jorgen ran across an article about it, he suggested we try it.

We arrived at Harbin on a day temperatures were well over a 100, one of the hottest of the year. I was certain we had made a terrible mistake. What were we doing in this unbearably hot place when we could be enjoying the serene coolness of the coast? I suggested we leave immediately. I had never seen Watsu, had only listened briefly to my daughter's comments about how nice it was. I was not that interested. But Jorgen explained it had taken several calls for him to get an appointment. He was able to convince me to at least talk to Elaine Marie, who was scheduled to watsu me.

As I talked to Elaine Marie I felt a unique quality in her gentle voice, a hidden laughter, a depth of understanding, that finally convinced me to receive a Watsu. So, totally unaware and unsuspecting, and with some reluctance, on August 6, 1990, I was watsued by Elaine Marie onto a totally new path.

A First Watsu

After my session, to help me understand what was happening, Elaine Marie explained how her life had been changed by Watsu, how she had given up a career to move to Harbin to watsu and teach, how it is her spiritual practice. Many of the things she said that night, when the moon had risen, resonate with what I had experienced.

"By folding and embracing the body, in warm water, skin against skin, close to the breast, heart beat connecting with heart beat, fetal memories of total trust and bliss are reestablished."

"It is the return to a place of total comfort, devoid of concerns, of worries, of anxieties."

I am floating on water, my head cradled on an arm so lightly, I feel only the water's buoyancy. I keep my eyes open, trying to take in this new experience. My mind, trained not to lose a detail, takes in the deep blue sky amidst the dark bay leaves, the shadows of the fig leaves on the shining water ... My body falls and rises, falls and rises, each time sinking deeper, returning lighter to the surface ... In spite of my resistance to let go of the images surrounding the pool, an inner force calls me inside. I close my eyes...

I no longer know whether I float or am carried in arms turned into a cradle. I rock into infancy, feeling the fragrant breast of my young mother, plentiful in sweet milk. I no longer pretend to know what's real, what's happening now or then, all sense of direction lost as my body is turned, floated, lifted, moved, swirled in the water.

I need to know what's happening to me. Am I still alive, in the pool held by this unknown woman? How can someone I've never met before project such tenderness, such lovingness. The need to be reassured of the reality of all of it leads me to open my eyes. The pool is now engulfed in shadows. The sky no longer blue but cobalt, shimmering with the prelude of a full moon. How much time has elapsed? It feels like an eternity. My connection with the reality around me has expanded. I do not need my eyes and again close them softly.

How can I possibly accept this gift of love from someone I don't know, who doesn't know me? How can somebody love so totally, so unquestionably: is it she, or are these older hands that hold me now? My grandmother lifting me from the crib, as the sun rises, taking me into the dawn, misty with dew, to see the cows get milked. And now surprisingly, I'm not lying on the water any longer. I have been lifted, my head falling onto my knee suspended in the air. Taken upon my father's shoulders for a stroll on the beach. The strength of his muscles a firm pedestal while the breeze from the shore sprinkles my face with salty mist, cooling me off, tickling my nose...Yes, the ocean, its immensity is here, taking me in, absorbing me, dissolving me.

Yes. It is powerful to return to childhood, to retreat to the womb. But I am far beyond, lost in the immense eternity of the primeval ocean. No longer aware of my own separation. All boundaries lost in the water.

As I float and am floated, lifted, turned, I let go of all possible concern, all judgments, all predicaments. No longer do I question the tenderness of the arms that keep holding me. The gentleness of the hands that squeeze my arms, that pull my fingers. I accept the commitment of love. I accept this love, unexpected, unrequested, and overwhelmingly total, because I am myself love.

"Watsu is a full sensorial experience. It's the whole of the body feeling the caress of the water. As in the womb, the closest sound you hear is another heart beat."

"Watsu takes someone back to the primordial experiences of the womb."

"The full awakening of the senses contribute to open your heart in receptivity to the love being bestowed on you."

After the First

At the ocean

As we left Harbin, Jorgen and I traveled, as planned, for several days on the Mendocino coast. I have always been a passionate lover of the ocean, but now I found I had a new connection to water, to all of nature. Trees, friendly companions of my childhood, took on new characteristics. The Watsu experience was forever in my mind. I realized I was walking with a new lightness. I was seeing the world with new colors. Something had happened within.

Effects continuing

But how to explain it? Was it a portentous interlude, an instant as brief as a glimpse of a rainbow, a ray of moonlight on the water, the sun on the emerald chest of a hummingbird? For a while I tried to continue my life as if nothing had happened, fulfilling the requests of my always full calendar. Speaking engagements took me to Williamsburg, to Houston, to Washington, DC., to Dallas. But the memory of the experience instead of fading became brighter. My dreams took on a Watsu quality. I would wake up not knowing if I was on a bed or on the water. Inadvertently, effortlessly, I lost some excess weight. I felt lighter, healthier, cheerful. People began to remark on my new softness. My own daughter commented: "I have never seen you being so comfortable in your body."

Called back

Yet it didn't occur to me to return to Harbin. I felt I had experienced a miracle, one which would be impossible to replicate. At the same time I was so intrigued by the experience that I kept contacting Elaine Marie to thank her for it. Finally she asked why didn't I return. The only time I could was a Saturday, between my flight back from a week as Visiting Author at the University of Texas, and a trip on Sunday to Los Angeles to deliver a keynote speech. I have never been too fond of driving and Harbin was a 3 hour drive each way, but I didn't want to refuse Elaine Marie's invitation to come to the drop-in Watsu class she teaches in the morning. I left home at 4 am.

A moment's hesitation

I parked the car to walk up to the pool, but for a moment I couldn't move. I was paralyzed by the conflict between wanting to reencounter the place where I had been spiritually renewed and fearing that I would lose the magic of that first experience.

The drop in class

It so happened that I was the only one to show up for her 'drop in' class. This seldom happens, but when it does Elaine Marie offers the sole student the option of receiving a Watsu. I welcomed the opportunity to be cradled and rocked into that space I remembered so fondly from my first Watsu, but still had some underlying fear it wouldn't be quite the same. It was and it wasn't. My surprise was the way it differed. With my greater level of surrender, my body became more receptive, the pleasure more exquisite, and the connection to the Universe, to the spiritual, happened almost immediately. The return to the womb was clear, but it was more than a place of trust and well-being. It was a place of love in which we know the connectedness of all the cells of our body, our unity.

Watsu of forgiveness

As I lay cradled in Elaine Marie's arms, on the steps of the warm pool, an immense sense of forgiveness arose in me. Any wrong doing, any mistake, any absurdity, any harm ever caused to me was being dissipated, eliminated from my body, from my mind, from my spirit. Just as I had melted into Love during the first Watsu, now I dissolved into forgiveness. Any feeling of resentment, pain or fear of suffering at the hand of another human being was replaced by a total loving of others. The often repeated "as we forgive those who trespass against us" became an overpowering existential experience, all of me turned into an act of total forgiveness.

Watsus stored

One of the extraordinary consequences of the Watsus for me has been how they are retained within me, long after the experience. They are stored as a physical or kinetic memory, as well as emotionally, and surface again, in their entirety and wholeness at different times.

Ovule

This second Watsu of forgiveness made itself manifest again much later during a Quantum Light Breathing meditation that Elaine Marie introduced me to. While sitting, focusing on the breath, I was jolted by a strong current of energy. My body jumped upward. I was returned to the experience of the second Watsu, to being in touch with the Womb, but this time I was ovule. In its diminutiveness, all life was contained. I curled up on the floor, quietly, contentedly contemplating this small form of life, expanding, expanding, expanding.

Rebirthing

When in the past people mentioned Rebirthing, I felt that I had, on my own as a writer, accessed memories of infancy. Even before I heard of Rebirthing, I wrote a description of my passage through the birth canal, my sadness on hearing my mother scream, my pain on hurting someone so nourishing, and my first encounter with the air at the end of the ordeal. I considered myself beyond any need for Rebirthing. Now I found myself spread out on the floor, giving birth to my own self, with the same contractions my body brought children into the world, with the same joy that graced the birth of my last child, giving birth to a self I had no idea had been waiting so long to be born.

A successions of Watsus

A successions of Watsus unfolded. The process continues. After the first, the Watsu of Unconditional Love, and second, the Watsu of Forgiveness, the third, the Watsu of Belonging, created in me a sense of total harmony with existence. In the fourth Watsu, Elaine Marie, rather than cradling me against her bosom, worked mostly from my back. As she pushed and pulled my body over the water, I dissolved into the water, into a deep understanding, not emotion, but a quietness, a serene all encompassing awareness. This transcendental Watsu brought me to peace, to a connection with the 'superior intelligence' that creates the Universe. It awoke a sense of clarity and of knowing, without effort or constraint. Aware that I was naming the Watsus, Elaine Marie chose to name this the Watsu of Gratitude.

Spiritual practice

Elaine Marie's spiritual practice of Watsu entails surrendering to each person in her arms with a devotion, with a love as unconditional as what the divine mother feels for each one of us. Guided by that love, each of her sessions is unique. Each is an improvisation, a dance to a new music, its flow and rhythm appropriate to the emotional and spiritual state of the person in her arms.

Eye contact

Our sixth watsu was a delicate dance of intimate sharing. We maintained more eye contact than previously, an eye contact that was in itself a form of dancing. As she made me soar, and turn, and dance joyfully on the water her eyes kept inviting me to mirror my happiness, my understanding, the supreme joy of existence. As I dissolved into her eyes, I found myself in Lightness.

Dancing toward the stars

As I closed my eyes, and let go into that lightness previously found in hers, I experienced a plenitude of being as never before. I had never felt as whole, as total, as free, as light, as happy, as truly, really me and yet free from ego or boundaries as I merged into the Oneness of love and light. And then, as I reached the total bliss of merely being, she began a dance toward the stars. By stretching my arms and pulling my body out of the water, making me gloriously free, she thrust me up to the sky and through the spiritual extension so powerfully taking place in me, I let go of my boundaries becoming truly one with the Universe.

Watsu of Tenderness

Elaine Marie named this the Watsu of Tenderness, because for her, tenderness had been the most prevalent feeling. I could not but concur, it had been for me the Watsu of Reaching for the Stars, the Watsu of Pleasurable Being, but unquestionably that connection with existence had taken place through her infinite tenderness.

Watsu of Sharing

The seventh is an appropriate Watsu to turn this account away from my individual experiences, which continued to unfold through many more wonderfully unique Watsus, to the new direction my life began to take as I learned to share Watsus with others. The seventh was the Magic Watsu, the Watsu of Sharing.

Learning to Watsu

Difficult learning

Elaine Marie had said that giving a Watsu was an even greater joy than receiving; and an even greater joy was teaching others to share it. From the beginning I felt the urge to learn to give back what I had received. Although Watsu is simple to learn, to me it seemed a gigantic task. From my childhood I have been physically uncoordinated. Gym classes were the nightmare of my youth. Not being able to dance was a perennial embarrassment in a family and culture where dancing is prevalent. Unable to draw or sew, to cook or do anything with my hands, except type, I had a very prolific academic and intellectual life, but felt totally overwhelmed by the idea of doing anything physical.

The art of teaching

Yet Watsu touched me so deeply it was unbearable to think I could not learn it. To my great fortune, Elaine Marie understands the urgency to learn and give Watsu which over-comes those who experience it. With infinite patience she set out to teach me. I have spent a lifetime observing teachers, and teaching how to teach. In this long career, in which I have had the opportunity to interact with exceptionally good educators, I have never met anyone more gifted in the art of teaching than Elaine Marie. Not only is she able to demonstrate and describe with great preciseness and insight the nuances of the process, but she is able to read inside her students, to understand their strengths and limitations, and to build their self-confidence and sense of worth as she patiently guides, over and over , until perfect mastery is achieved.

Being

In my case, she chose to focus on the aspects of Watsu that are not necessarily constrained by the physical movements. By insisting that Watsu is more "about Being than Doing," she enabled me to begin where I could: opening my heart to the person in my arms. As I learned to focus on another human being, to connect with their breath and their heart, to forget myself and to stand aside, in order that the experience could be fully theirs, while at the same time remaining totally present, in constant awareness of their needs, in full worship of their being, I began to realize that Watsu is indeed a form of life.

Staying in the place of touch

On teaching me the Shiatsu pressure points, Elaine Marie pointed out that while I was pressuring a point she felt that I was already focusing on the next. "It does not feel good to me if you know where your fingers are going next. As you press you must be there, at that point, as if the whole universe were reduced to that one place on the body where your thumb is pressing." As I tried to follow her directions, I became aware of how prevalent it has been in my busy life to be constantly preoccupied with the next task, and never truly totally in the present. How many times have I interrupted a student, convinced that I knew exactly where his questions were leading, and offered the solution that would allow us to move on, rather than truly listening? On shifting my attention to the present in Watsu, I began shifting my attention to the present in the rest of my life.

Listening to the body

"Listen to what the body wants, to what the body needs," Elaine Marie would say, while I would look in bewilderment at the body in my arms. Where does one begin listening to a body? How could I know what a body wants unless somebody told me specifically with words? Having always been involved in verbal communication, this listening to silence seemed the most demanding of tasks. Yet, wasn't part of the magic I had experienced the fact that Elaine Marie could so fully satisfy what my own body wanted, even when I wasn't even aware of what that was? Was not listening to the silent voices of bodies somehow connected to what had been my intellectual and political pursuit for years, to my own quest to "listen loudly", as one of my students had said, "to the unheard voices of the oppressed and silenced?"

Being present

"Be fully present. Do not allow anything in your mind, except your love for the person you hold in your arms. In this moment, in this instant, there is nothing else in the Universe. Disappear, do not intrude, respect, hold in awe, worship. Dare to love. Allow yourself to be consumed by love." Almost contradictory, and yet complementary, these directions to Watsu from Elaine Marie became directions to life.

Releasing the body

"As you fold the body into the accordion position, give the person a sense of her full being, and of her limits; as you hold her folded in your arms, claim her, and offer her your unconditional love and support. And now, as you release the body fully onto the water, let her experience the possibilities of her expansion, let her go, release her unto the Universe, step aside." These constant movements of Watsu, the contrast between holding, nurturing, caring, and releasing, letting go, restoring the person to full responsibility of caring for herself or himself, began to manifest in all of my life.

The Absolute

Of course, this did not all happen instantaneously, but was a process unfolding. One day as I watsued her, Elaine Marie made me aware that I had not yet gotten rid of my tendency to think and plan ahead in the Watsu. She very specifically said, "When your hand is moving up my spine, I need to know that the hand is where it is, and that at that moment, there is no past and no future. You do not know where the hand is going, because if you do, then I will feel it. But if you stay with the hand, there at a precise spot, with no thoughts in your mind of where the fingers are going, then you will be totally in the present, and the present will become eternity; I will experience the Absolute."

Changes

It was a hard lesson for someone who had lived trying to get the job done, moving right along, for someone intrinsically impatient as I had always been. Yet, as I practiced the deep meditation of staying fully focused on each moment, on each gesture, on each movement, I began to discover 'the experience of the moment' translating to other areas of my life. I began to write with more awareness. It became easier to pay attention to each sentence, to each word. I found myself producing more and producing more joyfully.

Flowers

When Elaine Marie speaks of surrendering, she speaks of the way she lives her daily life. For months she cultivated begonias on her deck. The bulbs she planted in the spring took a long time to bud, and longer yet to bloom. From visit to visit, I saw the buds grow under her patient care ... and the joy with which she welcomed each yellow flower when they finally started to open. But one day I stopped by and there was nothing but broken stems in the pots. There was a sad but tender smile on her face as she said: "I surrendered my flowers to the Universe, in the hunger of the deer. And now, part deer, they are still alive, playing and moving close to my deck instead of sitting on it."

Moving

Slowly, these experiences sank into me. I realized that much of the material reality that I had enjoyed previously meant very little, that the joy I found in the warm pool, as I melted with another heart, into the One Heart, was unsurpassed, and I moved to Harbin.

Return to nature

At no time has there been a sense of sacrifice nor deprivation in this change of life style, but on the contrary, the glory of living here is unsurpassed. I rediscovered the everyday excitement of nature: rather than collecting figurines of lady bugs as I used to do, now I could marvel at a lady bugs colony. The sounds of birds, crickets and running creeks have substituted those of landing planes and freeway traffic. I can rejoice in deer and hare, in raccoons and eagles, in quails and foxes.

Taking Watsu with me

Leaving

When I started living at Harbin every return to the city, where I continue to work, was an ordeal. It felt contradictory and painful to leave the newly found haven. Until I realized that what I had found lived inside of me. Wherever I go I can take it with me.

Watsuing my audience

The energy of Watsu enters my public speaking. As I face an audience, I feel the urge to take each and everyone in my arms and somehow I do. As I propose known concepts, and talk of familiar experiences, I fold up my audience as into the accordion position, their heads resting tenderly on my shoulder, while I claim them, and then as I present the challenges, the urgencies, the needs, I release them, the full body extended, returned to the water, acknowledging their own personal strength to cope, to find solutions, to be.

Listening without an answer

My students find me more attentive, more able to listen. I recognize that many times before in the urgency of wanting to be useful, I tried to anticipate what people were telling me. I had an answer ready. Now, I know each person is unique, and so is her or his process. I do not try to anticipate an answer, I merely listen as I would listen to a body on the water. And I truly hear.

Speaking about Watsu

As I have lost my fear of judgment by others, I have begun to speak about Watsu, only to discover that many of my academic friends are open to the experience. In fact I seldom need to bring up the topic, since those who know me ask about the transformation they perceive.

Watsu, dry and wet

I have taken Watsu with me in my travels. The 'dry' Watsu of the newly found attentiveness, of the heightened awareness, of the way I watsu audiences of up to several hundred people at the same time. But also the real Watsu. Hot tubs, hotel swimming pools, rivers, ocean, outdoor pools, any body of water will do for me. I am fully aware that the temperature of the water is the single most important element for successful Watsus, for allowing the maximum relaxation and therefore the longest non-interrupted Watsus. Yet, among the many things I am grateful for to Elaine Marie, I thank her for teaching me that time is a totally arbitrary concept, and that when it comes to Watsu, by working slowly deeply, with utmost concentration, time can be defeated, and eternity can be reached in a few minutes.

Earth Mother

I have watsued in Spain, in Mexico, in Miami, Philadelphia New York, Dallas, Houston, El Paso, Albuquerque, Tucson, Atlanta, and throughout California. I have watsued my own relatives, friends, and total strangers. In Southern California I watsued a young man in a hot tub, a friend of a friend of a friend, who had just attempted suicide and was caught in a deep depression. He wrote me a poem afterwards:

> Earth Mother.
> Unfolding Wisdom.
> Passage unto the Heart
>   of soul.
>   Embrace
>   of forgiveness
> I am of you
>   effortlessly
> born of the Womb.
> I am cleansed.

Inner City

Institute of educators

A few weeks ago I participated in a week long institute of educators concerned with social transformation. This year's institute took place at a spa near Palm Springs in Southern California. I made myself available to the group to teach Watsu at the few times (lunch and dinner hours) that the demanding schedule allowed. To my delight, several of the participants decided to learn. We made the best of the existing facilities, sometimes using the large hot tub, sometimes the swimming pool.

High school students

The highlight of the institute was a group of inner city high school students one of the participants brought to interact with us. The teacher had been offering his students, who were from very deprived socio-economic conditions (mostly Hispanics), the opportunity to reflect upon their own social reality, the issues of racism and prejudice, the significance of education, and the possibilities of a college education. All of this sounds very simple and logical, but unfortunately this is not the usual classroom practice. As a matter of fact these students and their teacher have suffered retaliation for being critical and outspoken. The participants of the institute had been very moved by the honesty and authenticity of the students and their willingness to face critically the complex reality of drugs, gangs, street violence, uprootedness, racism and multiple forms of oppressions that have surrounded their young lives.

Some questions

One morning, during one of the sessions in which I was not a speaker, I went to the pool to give a private Watsu session that had been requested by one out-of-state participant. While I watsued her in the shallow area of the pool, the kids were noisily playing at the deeper end. Toward the end of the Watsu they slowly approached, one by one, so that when I left the person, by now in a deep trance, resting on the steps of the pool, the kids were encircling me with several questions: "Is she asleep?" "Has she fainted?" "What did you do to her?" "What is this?"

An unexpected Watsu

I gave them a cursory explanation, believing that their interest would wane. But it didn't, so I asked if any of them would like to try it. A young woman rather reluctantly accepted, while the rest looked on rather skeptically. To me it was very moving. It was evident that there was a great deal of tension held in her young body and a surprising willingness to let go. When after a few minutes I brought her back to her feet there were loud exclamations of surprise from the kids: "Hey man, what did you do to her? Look at her face. It's glowing. There's light in her face, see that?" But their exclamations were silenced by the girl who herself exclaimed: "Hey you guys, you better try this. This is really unique. This is out of this world."

All participate

With her encouragement I organized a small class. Initially there was some resistance from the boys: "It looks motherly," one commented. I explained that Watsu was originally created by a man, that men do practice Watsu, that there is a nurturing quality in all of us. Finally all, except the four tallest boys, were willing to participate. And even those four, sometime through the class surprised me by joining in.

Depth of love

They had no difficulty learning the movements, but the extraordinary experience was to see their faces fill with tenderness towards each other as they discovered the deep joy of taking full responsibility for another human being in their arms. "If only I could do this to my mother," a girl exclaimed after I floated her using her as my model. "I need to be able to give this to my mother. She would be a different person," she added. Later, having reflected on the experience, she came back to tell me with great insight that she was going home a changed person. Now she would be able to see her mother with a new light. "I know I will not feel hurt by her anymore in the same way. I will keep remembering that what happens to her is that she has never been held like this. It will be easier to love and forgive her, knowing the depth of love she has missed out on in life."

Another girl exclaimed: "We need this. We need a club to do this. If we could experience this and help others experience it, who would need drugs?" As I gathered with them in a circle in the pool, after our few classes, I tried sharing with them what Elaine Marie always shares in her classes: "Once you have experienced this, you understand the space of vulnerability that is created for the person that you hold in your arms. It is necessary to respect that space." As I began to explain that Watsu is a very sensuous experience, and that it is possible that sexual feelings may arise, one of the boys, opening his arms, to encompass the whole group in his statement, just burst: "No worry, Man, this is sacred we are talking here, sacred..."

Watsu is expansive. Now my dream of an education that empowers students to take responsibility for their own personal life and for the collective transformation of the social reality to create a just, equitable, ecologically sound world of peace and respect, where individual and ethnic differences are celebrated, includes a Watsu class.

There are innumerable ways to access unconditional love. We live on a planet of diversity. There is not a tree, but madronnes, and walnuts, palms, ferns, oaks. There is not a flower, but roses and irises, violets, carnations and daisies. Each individual has her own path, his own journey. After a rich and fruitful life I have been given the gift of serenity, of inner peace. I have been shown a way to drop boundaries and melt with my fellow human beings into the eternal love of the One Heart. And, more importantly, I have been given a way to show others, how they, too, can let the waters in which they cradle and rock each other wash out everything but love.

WATSU II

Soft as petals your arms allow old memories, old frustations, and pains to dissolve in the water as the fears from the past become, through the power of love, the joyful recognition of the wholeness of being...

In morning ray
the water lily
opens
and sways
a white cloud
above the water
a flower that takes
decay
from under the river
up into the light...

CHAPTER IX

REBONDING THERAPY

A process

Rebonding Therapy is a process that integrates a series of bodywork sessions with movement meditations which a recipient can practice between sessions. Five forms of bodywork (three on land and two in water) are introduced in a way that their gradually increasing levels of nurturing non-sexual intimacy can best help the recipient heal his wound of separation, rebond to his oneness and be free in his separateness.

A continuity

Typically five sessions are scheduled. Half of each two hour session is bodywork. The other half is spent learning Movement Meditations which help maintain the effects of the bodywork. These can be practiced at home with the help of a video or audio tape. This practice, and the opportunity to discuss the continuing effects of previous sessions, provide a continuity within which the maximum potential of each form can be realized.

The five sessions

The first session's Co-Centering Shiatsu focuses on freeing the breath. Its Movement Meditation centers and harmonizes the 'breath' with the way the body moves in waves. In the second session a Watsu is given which focuses on freeing the body. The recipient is taught ways to free his own body in water. The third session's Tantsu focuses on opening the heart. Its Movement Meditation focuses on stretches that get us in touch with the streaming of the meridians. The fourth focuses on letting go into the joy and playfulness of a Free-flow Watsu. The concluding session, and its Freeform Tantsu, celebrate how all our centers connect, and how our connection to others is our connection to that which connects all. Its Movement Meditation focuses on connecting our chakras in ways that recreate the cycle of creation imprinted in our bodies.

Spiritual healing

On completing the process, besides whatever physical healing the body receives from this powerful bodywork, and whatever emotional clearing is reached, there is a spiritual healing. Rebonded to our oneness, freed from looking in others for what we miss in ourselves, we are free to be with others.

Healing the Wound of Separation

Connected and separate

One of the most powerful moments in a Rebonding session is when, after holding someone closely for up to an hour, we remove our hands and feel how, though we are no longer touching, we are still connected ... connected and separate. This connection that both feel, is not attachment, but the opposite. It is the ground of our freedom. It is returning to our original bond ... and our original separation. It is re-separating without the painful, disturbing, devastating dis-connections of separations that leave a wound, or rather, reopen the wound that reopens each time we are abused or betrayed or rejected. It is the same wound that reopens when others attach to an earlier self we need to separate from to grow. All growth is separation. Birth, itself, is separation. The more complete and loving the bonding immediately following it, the freer we can be when we make the necessary subsequent separations. In that moment at the culmination of a Rebonding session, the bond and the freedom are as simultaneous as in the moment of our original separation from the divine, a moment filled with the knowledge that we carry the divine out into our part of creation. The wound is the loss of that knowledge.

The wounded wound

The wound, and our attempts to hide it, affects all our relations with others. The more cut off we are from our oneness, the more likely we are to use others (and ourselves) as objects. . The less able we are to accept our separateness, the more likely we are to seek and conform to groups whose prejudices against outsiders create a false oneness, a oneness of wound.

Heal thyself   Traditional therapies try to make us face the wound by reliving events that add to it. In contrast, transpersonal Rebonding Therapy is a return to that oneness, the original loss of which is the source of the wound. This return is easier when it is made with another who came from that same place, who uses our help as much as we use theirs to return. We are each other's guides. We are all teachers, teaching each other to be with one another without intention, without ego, that false separateness that is the ignorance of our oneness. We are all healers. And the ancient prescription for the healer, "Heal thyself," steps beyond its usual interpretation as something we must do before trying to heal another. Instead it becomes the way itself

No Cause

Duality   The rebonded state cannot be reached by mind alone. The mind, when it is separated from the body, is doomed to duality. One of its basic dualities is cause and effect. The mind is continually looking for causes. There is no limit to the number of causes it could find for our debonded states. It will never find the cause. There is no single cause. If there were it would probably be the mind itself. But everything our parents and our culture have done to raise and acculturate us, and make us dependent on our institutions, are part of the cause. The cause does not exist in the past alone. It is all around us. The effect is the cause. This is in no way meant to be construed as a value judgment. The world is. And the world includes openings into transformation as profound as that achieved through Rebonding.

Unique among therapies   Rebonding Therapy may be unique among therapies in that it does not pretend to show people the cause of their problems. It does not attempt to make them relive their traumas. There is no screaming out of repressed rage or grief. No past life, no misaligned star is brought up. The balance of the organs is not questioned. Milk and chocolate are not blamed.

Addiction to cause   It is important to help free people from their addiction to cause, their habit of looking for someone who has the answer. If you cater to that need and come up with a diagnosis, you become their co-dependent. If, rather, you are with them in a way that helps them get in touch with their own oneness, you help free them from their addiction to cause. In oneness there is no cause.

Specific problems   This is not to deny that people have used, and will continue to use, the different forms of bodywork in this book as parts of therapeutic processes that deal with specific problems that have specific causes. Bodywork as powerful as this can facilitate many kinds of processes, including hypnotherapy, but such use should not be confused with Rebonding Therapy.

To truly be with others   The Rebonding therapist must free himself of the tendency to see people as products of causes. If your vision is limited in that way, it is impossible to truly be with others. If you know the oneness in yourself, that is what you see in others.

On Giving a Series of Sessions

Options   The five session series is sequenced to gradually introduce the non-sexual intimacy that is fundamental to Rebonding Therapy. Give your client the option to proceed slowly, to repeat levels as many times as needed before going on to the next.

The process   The sessions alternate bodywork on land and in water. This makes it easier for those who have limited access to a pool. There are three Movement Meditations on land. A new one can be introduced each time you work on land. These are available on both video and audio cassette that the client can purchase, as well as this book that has readings at the end of this section designed to prepare him for each session. In introducing the meditations you could follow the video with your client, pressing the pause button whenever you notice your client needs assistance, or when he needs time to explore movement further. These meditations are meant to be paused, and it is important to set the example.

The practice at home   A series of two hour sessions gives you the opportunity to receive feedback as to what were the long term effects of the previous session, and how the daily practice of the meditations went. The practice at home between sessions can be done cumulatively, i.e., after the second meditation is learned it can be practiced in sequence with the first, and the third proceeded by the first two.

Feelings that come up   Because you are working with a dance like flow that resonates with the flow of the energy being released, it is preferable to not play any background music during these sessions. It is also important to not interrupt the flow when an emotional release is occurring (unless he insists on stopping). It is better to help the person learn that whatever feelings come up can be carried along in the flow without detracting from the sense of completion and peace that comes at the end of the session. If he desires to share his experience afterwards, welcome it, but avoid any kind of analyzing or diagnosing that will separate him from the immediacy of what he is experiencing, an immediacy to which he needs to be rebonded.

Session I

Co-centering   Find out what expectations he has and what conditions require special attention or caution. Give him a complete co-centering Zen Shiatsu paying special attention to how it is opening his breathing. After separating, allow him time to assimilate the after affects of the session. Listen to any feedback he has to give. Have him stand up and lead him through the first meditation movement. Focus on how much he is letting the breath lead him into each movement. Help him find the most comfortable positions for his body. Arrange to have him meet you at the pool for the next session.

Session II

Watsu   Discuss the effects of the previous session and the Movement Meditation. This is his first Watsu. Have him first practice the Water Breath Dance. Give him an expanded Transition Flow, returning throughout to the breath rocking. If appropriate, the fourth section of the transition flow can be included, or it can be postponed until the next session in the pool. Practice sinking and Wai Chi with him. Teach him how to float. Tell him to continue practicing the first session's Movement Meditation at home, but to pause when he is lying on the floor to return to what it felt like floating and being watsued, to let his body move on the floor as it moved in water.

Session III

Tantsu   Discuss the effects of the previous sessions and the Movement Meditation. Depending on the amount of time left after this discussion, you could begin by doing the first meditation together. Starting with the Face Down position, give him a complete expanded Tantsu. Lead him through the second Movement Meditation. Show him how, when he reaches the place where he is lying on his back, he can pause the tape or video and explore the feeling of being in water.

Session IV

Free Flow   Discuss the effects of the previous sessions and Movement Meditations. Give him a complete Free Flow Watsu. If he can float well, show him some of the stretches that he can incorporate. Tell him to explore more water movement when he is lying on the floor in the second Movement Meditation, feeling the wave motions, letting his body become water.

Session V

Free Form   Discuss the effects of the previous sessions and the Movement Meditation. Give him a complete Free Form Tantsu. Lead him through the final Movement Meditation. Tell him that he can follow up the five sessions with a session in any one of the forms he has experienced.

To Those Receiving Rebonding

The effects

You are about to begin a process that can have a profound effect on the way you feel in your own body, and on the way you feel with others. You will receive five different forms of bodywork, two of which are done in warm water. All five coordinate stretching with releasing blockages in accupoints and chakra centers. All are done in dance like flows to the rhythm of the energy being released (no outside music will be played). The effects of this can be very tangible. This work can help normalize the functioning of every system in the body. It can help revitalize skin, muscle and other connective tissue. It can help open joints and increase their range of motion. The work, at times, can be quite deep, but it should not be painful. If at anytime you feel a stretch or pressure start to exceed the intensity that feels good, say something. Feedback is always welcomed.

New limits

Your body will be learning new limits, and new ways to move, and new ways to be held. The nurturing holding, the way your body is cradled during much of this bodywork, the bonding without 'attachment', will help you overcome barriers to non-sexual intimacy. Many feel a very deep level of connection and oneness in this work. The deeper that level, the freer you can be in your separateness. The less one feels that connection, the more one seeks it in others. The more you feel that connection and oneness in your own body, the freer you can be with others.

The flow

Our bodies carry memories of past abuse and trauma. It is common, as different parts of our body are handled and stretched, to have all kinds of feelings come up-- sorrow, rage, grief, desire... Do not be dismayed, or ashamed. There is no need to hide or suppress anything. Be aware of whatever feelings come up, and let them be part of the flow the whole body is feeling. What better way to learn to accept such things in the flow? This work almost always leads to a real sense of completion, of peace, at the end. Afterwards you are free, but not required, to share whatever happened to you. The focus of this work is on the flow, and the oneness felt in it, rather than on analysis, interpretation or diagnosis.

Be

Wear loose cotton clothing to your sessions on land, so that you can be fully stretched. All the work on land is done in clothing. Since oil is not used, clothing does not interfere in any way with this work's holding, pressing and stretching. Each of the five forms entails a slightly higher level of non-sexual intimacy. Any one of the forms can be repeated as many times as you like before going on to the next level. Before each session read the section below relating to it. A rule of thumb during the bodywork is "Do nothing. Just Be." Be in your body. Everything is in your body. Don't try to breathe, or not breathe, in any special way, or assist in stretches and movements. Enjoy.

Practice at home

You can purchase either a video or an audio cassette to follow along and practice Movement Meditations each day at home. The practitioner will go through each level's new movements during the second half of your sessions. These provide a way to explore further the centering, the breath opening, and the flows of energy that the bodywork facilitates. These help you keep in touch with that part, or rather that wholeness of your body, that is the most immediate, and the most creative, long after the series is completed.

I Freeing the Breath

Co-centering

Your first session will be Co-centering Zen Shiatsu. The practitioner will be connecting and reconnecting, throughout the session, heart and body centers, and, at the end, mind center. While one hand (or elbow or knee) is leaning into a series of points, the other will stay in one place and provide constant support. The way this work is done to the rhythms of your breathing, helps free your breath to open into more and more of your body. Enjoy that opening. Shiatsu's pressing the traditional points of acupuncture, and its stretching of the meridians that connect those points, helps balance the flow of 'chi' energy in your body. Enjoy the feeling of this flow throughout your body. This is your own healing energy.

II Freeing the Body

Watsu   Before receiving your first Watsu, let the practitioner know whatever expectations or feelings you have about water, or if you have a tendency towards seasickness. As always give feedback if anything is uncomfortable. If you are disturbed by water going in and out of your ears, you can wear swimmer's ear plugs. Take care of all this before you start the Watsu, because once it starts, you may find yourself in a different world, where there is no sense of time. You may lose all sense of up and down. In the Basic Watsu, a very simple rocking is returned to again and again. This becomes a sort of ground that the other movements and stretches flow out of. The practitioner will use his own body to capture part of your body so that the uncaptured part can be more freely moved. You will feel your spine and body moving in ways that it never has before. Your body is being re-educated, learning greater and greater freedom. At the end, when you are at the wall and the practitioner lifts off his hands, feel how you are still connected and separate. Take your time. If you feel like it, let your body sink in the water and explore how freely it can move. Explore this same freedom when you are lying on the floor in the Movement Meditation.

III Opening the Heart

Tantsu   Instead of using his body to lean in with as in the first session on land, in Tantsu, the practitioner uses his body to cradle and support your whole body throughout the session. Much of the intimacy, and power, in this work is due to the support that all these forms, except Zen Shiatsu, provide the first chakra, which is in the perineum between the legs. This is a non-invasive support that occurs when you are sitting on someone's lap or knee while other parts of your body are being focused on. The first chakra is where our energy, at the bottom of the breath, returns into the void. It is the base of whatever rises up the spine. When it is shut down, there cannot be a complete opening of any other chakra. Tantsu effects all the chakras, particularly the Heart chakra, whose opening is facilitated by the constant nurturing holding.

IV Free Flow

In this second Watsu session, the movement becomes freer, more spontaneous than in the first session. If you are inflexible and difficult to float and move in the water, the moves in this session may not be very different than in your first session, but you will find this, and every session different. Do not come to any session with expectations. Just be in your body, experiencing what is happening at that moment.

V Free Form

In this final session you will find your body being held and rocked in some of the same positions as in the Tantsu as well as new ways. More than anything this is Watsu on land. Feel how the flow of this work breaks through the boundaries between land and water. You can do the same in your Movement Meditations and discover again and again the fluidity of movement that is creative.

After the Series

You can continue to practice at home the Movement Meditations, and further explore ways to center and free your body. You can return for a follow-up session in any one of the above five forms as often as is needed. A good way to continue growing with this work is to share it with others. Simple forms of both the work on land and the work in water are presented in this book and the videos that accompany it. Intensives and weekend workshops are also available.

CHAPTER X

CREATIVE MOVEMENT MEDITATIONS

Creative movement is the movement that arises spontaneously when we are most present in our body, when our body is most free. Because it is creative, there is no limit to the number of forms it can take. Its most basic form is that of the wave. Creative movement is internally generated. It comes from within and spreads freely through the body. It may or may not be externally visible. On the cellular level it is continuous. Its presence defines life. It can be manifested in swift vibrations rising up the spine, or in very slow undulations of our body. Emptying into the void at the bottom of the breath, getting in touch with the flows of our meridians, and connecting our chakras are ways to open ourselves up to creative movement. Water is ideal because it allows a greater amplitude of wave motion than being on land. Our bodies are made of water and they still have within them memories of all the forms of water experienced in our personal development and in the evolution of life. These can be accessed on land. The following opens with movement in water and then moves on to three Movement Meditations on land. If you are not in a pool, you can skip ahead to the meditations on land.

THE WATER WAY

The following presents ways you can explore the connection and freedom of your body in water. As with Watsu, the ideal place for exploring these comfortably and slowly, is in water the temperature of your body's surface. If the water is cooler, you may need to intersperse moments of faster, more active movement, to keep yourself from chilling.

The Water Breath Dance

Sinking and rising

There is a simple practice you can do in a pool to co-ordinate your breathing with your body's letting go in the water. Settle into water that is two thirds as deep as your height, your legs spread as wide as is comfortable, each foot staying in its place. As you breathe out let your body sink to whatever direction it wants (keeping your nose out). Feel how, as you breathe in, the water lifts you back up, and how, as you breathe out, it lets you back down. Notice any holding in your knees or elsewhere. When you breathe out, sinking, let go of it a little more. Notice how, at the bottom of the breath, there is a moment of total stillness, of emptiness, before the breath and the water start you back up towards the surface. Keep doing this until you feel one with your breath and the sinking and rising, until you feel it is the water breathing you up and down, until you feel one with the water, your partner, in this Water Breath Dance.

Sinking

*The stillness at
the bottom*

To be completely comfortable in water both sinking and floating should be as natural to you as your own breath. To explore sinking on a deeper level take three deep breaths and, blowing all the air out, let yourself settle to the bottom. Lying on your back do a series of swift abdominal contractions and then lie perfectly still. Feel how comfortable it is to lie on the bottom, and how long you can lie without breath (Don't try this in a crowded pool ... nor in a completely empty pool ... Have someone around in case you forget to come up). When you do come back up, do it slowly without rushing or panic, and, when your head comes out of the water don't gasp for air but breathe in naturally. Learning to lie on the bottom of a pool without fear may have further benefits. I remember the sense of empowerment the first time I lay quietly at the bottom not unlike what someone must feel after fire walking.

Wai Chi

Tai Chi in water

Water is ideal for slow, Tai-chi like movement. Our basic Water Dance, and the Watsu itself, is done in this spirit. Alone in the pool, as you sink into the Water Dance, let your body settle into and come back up out of the water. Each time your head goes under, let the completion of your body's movement bring your head back out rather than the desire to breathe, or the fear of running out of breath. When you do come up, take your time and breathe in slowly. See how completely your body's movements can be coordinated with your breathing without intention or fear. Explore how every movement leads to its completion and opens to another movement. Explore all the connections of movement.

Floating

Reservoir of air

The more body fat you have, the easier it is to float. Even those with a limited amount of fat can learn to float, if they practice controlling their breath and the tonus of their body. A way of breathing that can help you float is to always maintain a reservoir of air in your lungs by never completely emptying them. The tonus can be achieved by keeping your arms stretched up over your head and your legs straight, at the same time as you keep your whole body relaxed.

Three States

*Steel, rubber
and wood*

You can have someone else help you arrive at this state. Have someone stand beside you, one hand under the back of your head, the other under your sacrum while you lie back in the water, your arms straight up over your head. Imagine your whole body is as rigid as steel. Tighten every muscle in your body. Feel how heavy you are in the water. Next imagine your whole body is rubber, totally limp. Feel how your body would sink if someone wasn't holding you. Now imagine your whole body is wood, not the wood in a piece of furniture but the wood in a living tree. Feel the life of a tree from the tips of your toes all the way up to your fingertips. Feel the resiliency of wood, how different it is than the stiffness of steel and the limpness of rubber. Feel how much easier it is to float when you feel this extension of life throughout your body. At this point the person holding you can move down to below your feet and gradually remove support from under them.

Woga

Water is ideal for stretching, for Water Yoga. Depending on the available depths, this can be done standing, sitting and lying, as well as floating. If there is a bar, many stretches can be improvised at the wall. What follows is a sequence that can be done while floating in the state of tonus described in the previous section. Besides opening up those parts of the body being stretched, doing this while floating provides opportunities to explore extension in parts not being held in a stretch.

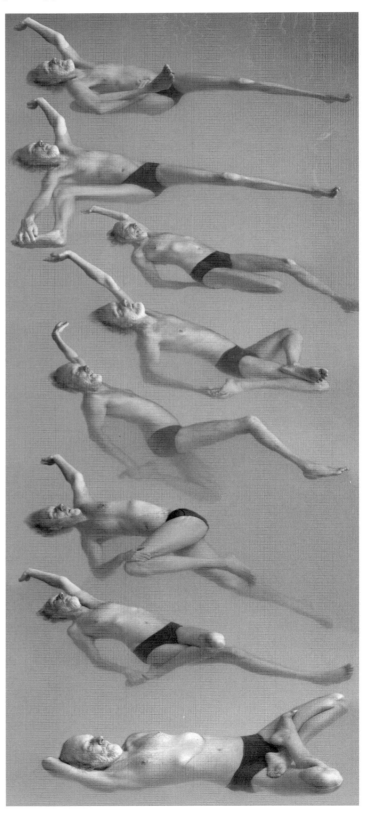

a. Leg Wrap

Float on your back, your arms up over your head. Move your right knee as near to the right side of your chest as possible. Hook your right elbow under it and place your right hand on your hara just below the navel. Float.

b. Pull Wide

Remove your right hand from your hara and hold your right foot, pulling your right leg straight. Feel how wide out your left arm and leg spread as you stretch the muscle down the back of your right leg.

c. Heel Up

Hold your right foot near the toes and press the heel of your right foot into your right buttock. Hold and feel the powerful straight line of extension up left arm and down left leg.

d. Flying W

Press your right foot up to the surface, lifting with your right hand under the inside of your right foot. Prop your left foot over your right thigh. Let your left arm curve up over your head. Float.

e. Pull Under

Slip your left foot off your right thigh as you reach under with your right hand and pull the left foot towards your right side. Let the rest of your body reach out in whatever way balances and amplifies this stretch.

f. Twist

Release the left foot. With your right hand pull your left knee across the top of your right thigh to twist stretch your spine.

g. Leg Over

Pull your left foot towards the side of your right hip, wrapping your left knee around your right thigh.

h. Lotus

If you are comfortable in lotus position, slide your left ankle over the top of your right leg. Reach down with your right hand and prop the other ankle over the top of the other leg. Float and explore movement in lotus. If you can hook your fingers behind your back, one arm under your head and the other under your waist, you will find yourself tied up in a way that supports your head and allows you to float freely.

i. Second Side

Float with your arms up over your head and repeat the mirror image of the above on the second side.

j. Knees Up

Wrap your upper arms (coming from between) around your knees to press them to your chest.

k. Feet pull

Hold your feet, the bottoms pressed together, with both hands and float.

l. Both Heels Up

Holding a foot in each hand, press their heels up towards your buttocks and float.

m. Shake Free

Straighten your legs and float, allowing vibration or shaking to work its way up your body in stronger and stronger waves. Notice how those waves' changing as they pass up your head and neck can lead you into a state of total ecstasy, how everything around you becomes brighter, and freer. As the undulations coming up your spine become stronger and stronger, be careful to not let your head jerk back so violently it strains your neck. If that becomes a danger, try accessing the same waves while standing (or kneeling) under water where your spine is vertical and your head has the support of the water.

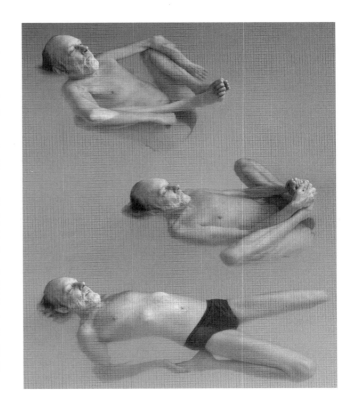

A Smile On The Face Of The Deep

Water out of water

Water is in our every cell. We came out of water. We have experienced water in all its shapes and forms. We know water. When we explore water within water we surrender and move in whatever way that particular body or form of water allows. When we explore water outside of water, we can explore all the forms of water and its movement that our body knows, wave, river, undertow, water spout, still pond. Water is shape changing. And so are our bodies. In Creative Movement all the states and forms we know from our own individual development, from the evolution of life, and from creation itself, can be accessed within our bodies.

Experiencing creation in our bodies

We begin out of what was before the beginning- the void, the Chaos that creation stories describe as a dark sea, as the Face of the Deep. Where we can most feel this in our own bodies is in the emptiness at the bottom of the breath, when, rather than following the breath out, we center in the emptiness left behind. This is the moment in the breath cycle when our diaphragm and our abdominal muscles have most completely relaxed, the moment before they become activated again as we breathe in. If we center and ground ourselves in this emptiness, there is no part of creation that we cannot experience rising up out of it, and returning back into it. The way of the breath, the way our bodies move to it, the way we empty into the void at the bottom of the breath, and are raised back up out of it in waves, is the focus of the first Movement Meditation. In the second we stretch our meridians and focus on the energy pathways in our body in a way that take us through another cycle of creation. A third creation cycle is experienced in the last meditation when we connect our centers or chakras. The three Movement Meditations can be each practiced separately, or as one long uninterrupted process. The more we experience creation, and its flows and centers, within our bodies, the more we will find our bodies opening to spontaneous creative movement. Feel free to spend as long as needed when this starts to happen. These meditations are as flexible and adaptable to individual needs as the bodywork in this book. If you are following this on video or audio cassette, have a pause button near at hand and use it whenever you are in a place where you feel the opportunity to further explore movement (or stillness).

When doing the following it is best to be in a room with a rug comfortable enough to lie on. Wear clothing loose enough to stretch in. When asked to sit, sit in whatever position is comfortable and best helps keep your back straight. If you are going to need a cushion, or a chair, have one near by.

BREATH AND WAVE

In the following you will stand, rocking your body to your breath, and explore how your breath and body become one. You will get down on hands and knees and explore how your body opens to the filling and emptying of the breath. You will sit and enter even deeper into that emptiness at the bottom of the breath, which is the void before creation (The Face of the Deep). You will explore the wave movement in your own body, which is the movement of life rising out of that void. You will explore the aquatic, the animal and the human dance. You will stand and hold in your hands the peace that is at the center. You will lie in the wave.

The Way of the Breath Rocking

The body's dance to the breath

Stand, legs spread as wide as is comfortable, shoulders relaxed, arms hanging loose to your sides, face and neck relaxed, hips and knees. Breathe out slowly, slowly settling into your body, your knees bending. Breathe in slowly straightening your legs. Feel how your body rises up as the breath fills it. Each time you breathe out let your body sink to whatever direction, and as deeply, as it wants. Each time you breathe in feel that rising up your spine, all the way up your body. Explore all the ways your body might want to sink as it lets go into the outbreath, as your breath empties and your body empties with it. Enjoy the sinking into that emptiness, and the rising up out of it each time you breathe. Your body is one with your breath. Gradually build up the pace of your breathing. Breathe faster and faster. Your body, rocking to your breath, sinks and rises faster and faster. Your arms start swinging by themselves to its rocking. Let them swing to whatever direction and as high as they want. Notice how it is your breathing that is rocking and swinging your body and arms. When it has reached a joyful, playful pace, when it is dancing free to your breath, gradually slow down your breathing. Slower and slower, your body rocking slower and slower. Slow it down until the rocking becomes totally internal, until your body is no longer visibly moving. Feel how there is still an internal sinking each time you breathe out, and a filling, a rising each time you breathe in. Feel how even in stillness there is an internal rocking, a sweet pulsing of the breath. Breath and body are one. *(Pause)*

The Way of the Breath Opening

Breathing in the stillness

Slowly get down on your hands and knees, spreading them as wide as is comfortable. Keeping your shoulders relaxed, and your arms straight, slowly rock forward as you breathe out, and back as you breathe in, but not so far back that any effort is required to rock forward again. Keep your neck relaxed. Each time you rock forward, feel the letting go in your center just below your navel. Each time you breathe in and rock back feel the rising up your spine. Continue rocking to the breath this way until it becomes totally automatic, until breath and body are one. Sit as far back between your knees as is comfortable. Place your elbows on the floor in front of your knees, your head dropped between them. Without moving externally, continue to feel the breath rising up your spine and emptying back into your center. Stay as open to this breath as a hollow tube. Feel how at the very bottom of the breath, there is an emptying all the way into the perineum, and how, from that point between your legs, there is a rising all the way up your spine as you breathe in. Enjoy the peace that comes with being open, with being one with the emptying and filling that breathes in the stillness. *(Pause)*

The Way of the Breath Emptying

Sitting

Sit in whatever position best helps keep your back straight and is comfortable. If necessary, place a cushion under your tailbone, or sit on the edge of a chair. Rest your hands, palms up, in your lap, one hand lying in the other, the tips of your thumbs touching. Relax face, neck, shoulders, back, sacrum, buttocks and the rest of your body. Feel how straight your spine can be without effort. Feel how as you breathe in, the filling rising up your spine, is a wave spreading out to all parts of your body. And how, as you breathe out, all those parts settle and empty into the center. Be aware of any part that doesn't empty as much as the rest and, the next time you breathe in, fill that part even more. As you breathe out, let it, let everything empty into the center.

The bowl at the base of the spine

Be aware of the whole area around the center, the navel-- the front, the sacrum-- the back, and the perineum-- the bottom. This whole area around the center is a bowl at the base of the spine. Each-time you breathe out, everything empties into that bowl ... and rises up out of it each time you breathe in. At the very bottom of the breath when everything has emptied into that bowl, for a moment, the bowl itself is empty. When everything has emptied into that bowl, the bowl empties into that point at the bottom, the first chakra. This is where our energy returns into the void, which is its most powerful state, because it is pure potential. At the bottom of each breath empty into that void. Notice what happens as the breath starts up your body again. Let whatever opens to it, open. Let whatever moves to it, move. Movement is life. And out of that stillness in the void comes all life. There is no part of your being that is not at this moment moving out of that stillness. Every bone, every muscle, every cell is moving, however slightly, wave upon wave. You are the Face of the Deep. Smile. *(Pause)*

The Way of the Wave

Crawling up in the animal

Every movement begins as a wave. Begin the waves that are your arms and legs, and get down on all fours, on hands and knees, a wave rocking your body into whatever shape it wants, rocking you back and forth. The waves bring you up onto your hands and knees and rock you, wave upon wave. Your spine, flexible, moves to whatever waves rise up out of the void and wash you up onto the shore. And that void continues to flow into whatever shape it rocks your body, into whatever animal crawls up out of that void, into whatever growl or laugh comes out of your throat. There is nothing that does not come out of the void, wave upon wave. *(Pause)*

Standing in the dance

When the void has completed its crawling up over the earth, let the wave lift you up to stand. Stand. Hold the area around your center, around your navel, in both hands. From the animal comes the human, human hands holding human center, human spine upright, but still flexible, still wavering in the waves that rise up. Feel the peace in your hands. Hold it in your hands as the waves rise through your body. Feel that peace in your center as the waves slowly move your arms out in front of you, as the waves rock and move your whole body, freer and freer, your spine moving, turning, spiraling in whatever waves rise up it. Everything is moving in waves. And however freely arms, legs, neck, head move there is still a unity, a oneness, a joy in the dance, a stillness. That peace is as much one with all these waves as is the particle in the waves of matter. Focus on the stillness in each wave as your arms lower, as your body's movement slows down and becomes still. Feel the inside of the waves, the hollow places under the waves, moving without movement in your body. Still. Stand still. Still dance. Still.

Lying in the wave

Slowly lower yourself to the floor and lie back, your arms spread out to the sides. Settle into the floor as into the waters of a warm ocean, its slow gentle waves slowly rocking your body in waves. There is no difference between whatever waves you feel within your body and whatever waves slowly lift and rock your body. They are all one wave. Your body and your breath and your rock are all one wave that goes on and on and on. There is no end to the wave.

MERIDIANS STREAMING

In the following you will stretch the meridians of the legs and explore how they connect us to the earth and the power we get from and return to the earth. You will stretch the meridians of the arms and explore how they open to the outside and protect the inside. You will get in touch with other energy pathways, our breathing and our senses, and how they also have a Yin and a yang flow.

Opening our Connections to the Earth

Yang flows down to the Earth

Stand, facing the center of the room, knees slightly bent. The breath pulses. It is oceanic. Movement from within goes out through the body in waves. Meridians are steady flows along the surface of the body. Stand still. Focus on the surface. One pair, the central meridians, flows up the back and down the front. It is a lake the other meridians flow out of as rivers, each bearing its share of our life force, their functions related to where they flow. There is a flow all the way down the front of your body. The meridian of the front begins just under the eyes and flows down chest, belly, legs, all the way down. We go out in front of ourselves to get food, our sustenance from the earth. There is a flow all the way down the sides of your body. The meridians of the side begin to the outside of the eyes and flow down both sides down shoulders, hips, ankles, all the way down. They have to do with deciding which way to go, this way or that, with our power, with how we use the energy we get from the earth. There is a flow all the way down the back. The meridian of the back begins to the inside of the eyes and flows up over the top of the head and all the way down the back, water flowing down the back, down the back of the legs. It has to do with elimination, with purification, with what we leave behind and return to the earth, or don't, and still carry on our back.

Front

All these meridians that start around the eyes, that flow down front, sides and back, flow down to the earth. Follow that flow down to the earth, all the way down. Get down on the earth. Get down on your knees and lean back, placing your hands on the earth behind you. Keep your arms straight. Keep hands and knees grounded, planted in the earth. Raise your hips higher and higher. Stretch the meridian of the front, the meridian of the earth. Arch it up as curved as the earth. Hold it as long, and stretched as high, as you comfortably can.

Side

Lower your hips and slide your legs out from under. Straighten and spread your legs out to the sides as wide as possible. Raise your hands up in the air. To stretch the meridian of decision and power, decide what side you're going to stretch toward. Decide and, keeping your chest facing forward and open, lean to that side. Feel the power opening, stretching the side you are leaning away from. Each time you breathe out feel the stretch open up more. Straighten up and lean to the other side. What you feel being stretched is the meridian of the green that grows out of the earth.

Back

Straighten, arms still up over your head. Bring your legs closer together, straightened out in front of you. Keep your back and arms and legs straight. Slowly swing forward to stretch the meridian of the back. Feel its stretch all the way down the back of your legs. This is the meridian of water. If we could let go of all that we carry, our backs would be water. On each outbreath sink a little deeper into the stretch. Do not rock but stay as you breathe in, and sink a little deeper as you breathe out, feeling it slowly open to its flow.

Lying in the flows

Slowly lower yourself back on the floor, arms out to the sides. Lie still and feel whatever flows these stretches have opened up in your body. *(Pause)* When you feel the flow down the front of your body, feel the earth in your body lying on the earth and its movements. When you feel the flow down the back, feel the water your body is spreading out over the earth, and its movement. When you feel the flows down the sides, feel the richness of new life watered and growing out of the earth, and its movement.

Growing out of the Earth

Grow out of the Earth. Slowly raise your knees and pull them to your chest. Hugging them to you with both arms, feel the roundness of the earth in your body. Lay your right arm out to the right, and keep your right shoulder on the ground, as you slowly lower your bent knees to your left and twist over the earth as slow as a vine. Pull your knees back up and hold them to you again. Lay your left arm out and slowly twist to your right. Continue rolling to the right until you roll up onto your knees, spreading them as wide as is comfortable. Rest your forehead on the earth. Keep your hands rooted in the earth you grow out of, as you straighten your arms, and raise your knees off the ground, your feet spread and rooted in the earth. Slowly walk your hands towards your feet as your legs straighten up, your waist still bending over the earth you grow out.

Inside and Outside

The Yin flow up and the Yang down

Each one of the three Yang meridians, whose flow you followed down the outside of your body, has a Yin partner that flows up the inner surfaces of your legs. Feel that flow up from the earth your legs are still rooted in. Keep your arms hanging toward the earth and slowly straighten your back vertebra by vertebra. Follow that yin flow up the inside of the legs, up through the hara, up to the area around the heart. This is the area where all the yin flows up the arms begin. When your back is straight let that rising Yin slowly raise your arms up in front of you. Feel that flow of Yin up their inner surfaces. When your arms are raised as high as the highest branches of a tree, reach up into the Yang and feel its flow down the outside of your arms. Each of the three Yin meridians in the arm has a yang partner that flows down the outside, down into neck and face where all the Yang meridians that flow down the legs begin. The Yang flow from Heaven to Earth, down the outside. The Yin flow from Earth to Heaven, up the inside.

Interchange between inside and outside

Spread your arms out at an angle midway between straight up and straight out, the angle which best opens your chest. Stretch them back to open the chest more and more. What is stretching now is the pair of meridians that have to do with the interchange between the inside and the outside. This is the stretch that opens this pair to the outside. Feel how open your lungs are. To stretch the same meridians to the inside, lower your arms and hook your thumbs behind your back. Pull your shoulders back. As you breathe out, bend forward at the waist and swing your arms, thumbs still hooked, vertical up over your back. Hold. Stretch the arms further forward each time you breathe out. Come up slowly and stand still a moment, letting your arms hang at your side. Feel the openness between the inside and the outside.

The deepest inside

There is a deeper inside. Raise and bend your right arm behind your head. Hold your right elbow with your left hand and pull it toward your left shoulder. This stretches the meridians that have to do with that deepest inside-- the heart. It opens them to the outside. Change arms behind your head and stretch your left arm toward your right shoulder, opening that side to the outside. To stretch the same meridians to the inside, lower your arms and, facing the center of the room, sit on the floor. Hold your feet in your hands and pull them into you as close as possible, the soles of your feet pressed together, your knees spread out and as close to the floor as possible. Surrender the straightness of your back. Round it forward, stretching your whole being around your inside, around that deepest center in your chest.

Surface

Sit up and cross your legs. Sit in whatever position best helps you keep your back straight. Raise your arms straight up, palms forward. Swing them back to stretch up their midline. The meridians you are stretching open to the outside now are the ones that have to do with the surface, with what protects that deepest center we stretched around before, and what comes to the surface from that center. To stretch the same to the inside, keep your back straight, cross your arms and pull your opposite knees without swinging them up.

Pathways All Around

The senses

Rest your hands on your lap, one in the other, palms up, thumbs touching. Sit, your back straight. Focus on the meridians' flows in your body. You have stretched the meridians in your legs that connect you to the earth and its power, and those in your arms that open to the outside and protect the inside. There are other energy pathways. Our senses reach out way beyond our arms. Our senses are energy pathways that also come in yin and yang pairs. With eyes closed focus on sight. Looking is yang. It is a going out, and seeing is yin. It is an accepting in. Behind closed eyelids, look. See. Listening is Yang, and hearing Yin. Listen. Hear. Touch is Yang, and feeling Yin. Without moving touch the space around your hands, the clothes around your body. Feel that space and the clothes on your skin. So much of the time we look without seeing, we listen without hearing, we touch without feeling. See. Hear. Feel. And the breath is an energy pathway. What rises as we breathe in is Yang, and what empties as we breathe out is Yin. Open up to the Yin at the bottom of the breath. Completely empty into that emptiness. It is our grounding place within. The more we ground in it the freer flow the central meridians, those that rise up the back and settle down the front, that lake that all the others flow out of. Still water.

CENTERS RESONATING

In the following you will explore how your energy centers can be connected in ways that recreate the creation cycle outlined in the Taoist canon, the Tao Te Ching. You will explore the ways your body spontaneously moves to the resonances established between the centers at each stage of creation. You will explore creation and how at the bottom of every breath we return to the moment before.

The Tao And The One Being Born

The void   Sit, hands in your lap, thumbs touching, a circle. As you breathe in feel the rising up your back, a wave spreading out to all parts of your body. As you breathe out feel how all those parts let go and settle and empty into the center. Be aware of the whole area around the center, the navel -- the front, the sacrum -- the back, and the perineum -- the bottom. It is a bowl at the base of the spine. Each time you breathe out, everything empties into that bowl. At the very bottom of the breath, when everything has emptied into that bowl, the bowl itself empties into the point at the bottom, the first chakra, which is where our energy returns into the void, which is its most powerful state because it is pure potential.

In the *Tao Te Ching* Lao Tzu says,

> The Tao gives birth to the One
> The One gives birth to the Two
> The Two gives birth to the Three
> And the Three to the Ten Thousand

The Tao   What you feel in that void at the bottom of the breath is the Tao, the undifferentiated, the mother of all beings. What you feel rising up your back as you breathe in is the Tao giving birth to the One. The One is your crown chakra, where you are one with everything. Empty into that void, into the Tao at the bottom of the breath, and feel how, as you breathe in, the One is being born all the way up your back, all the way up the back of your head, all the way up to that place of light, not a seeing light but a being light, a shining out to all sides. And as you breathe out, feel how all that light settles back down the front, as slow as snow falling, darkening as it empties back into the Tao.

The Deepest Heart Center

The continuous   We have been using our breath as a vehicle, but this rising up the back and settling down the front is a continuous cycle. And the Tao is continuous. And the One is continuous. Where we can most feel its continuity is midway between the rising and the settling, midway between the Tao and the One, at the center of that whole continuous circle, in the deepest center in the heart center.

Opening the heart

As you focus on this deepest center be aware of what your body is doing, or wants to do. This is our most personal, most private, most vulnerable center. Our bodies develop ways to protect it. Feel how your body protects it, maybe a tightening, a drawing in of your shoulders. Let it. But the next time you breathe out let all that protection and vulnerability and pain settle and empty back into the Tao. As you breathe in feel how open your heart center can be. Feel that openness in your arms. Slowly raise them and hold them out in front of you, a circle, your fingers almost touching, palms facing your heart center. Feel the openness of your heart center in your arms, arms that hold those you love. Let those arms and your torso freely dance that loving openness. *(Pause)* When it has fully opened, lay your two hands, one on top of the other, over your heart center, still holding its openness.

The Two

Heart and mind

Lay your hands on your knees, palms up. Just as there is a deep center in your heart, there is a deep center in your mind. Focus on these two at the same time. As you focus on these two, notice whatever movement, or tendency to move, there is in your body. Maybe a rocking from side to side, or a spiraling. As it moves so, notice how these two never come any closer together, and never move any further apart, but dance, forever maintaining the same distance. These are the Two that are born out of the One- Heart and Mind, Soul and Spirit, Yin and Yang. These are the two poles of all the meridian pairs that create and maintain the life of your body. Feel the wholeness of their flow from head to feet to heart, and from heart to hands to head. Feel what a beautiful creation your body is, a creation of the dance of Heart and Mind.

The Three

Body, heart and mind

The body has its own center on the surface, just below the navel. And the Heart has a center on the surface, the Heart Chakra. And the Mind has a center on the surface, the Third Eye. These are the three you face the world with, your strength, your love, your clarity. As you focus on these three notice whatever movement your body begins to make. Maybe a rocking forward this time because these are the three you face the world with. Notice how these three resonate together. It is not pulse nor flow but resonance that connects our chakras. But they are not always in harmony, in balance. Notice whatever balance there is between these three now.

The Ten Thousand

All we have said and done

Midway between the body center and the heart center, in the solar plexus, is the center of your will, of your actions, of your deeds. Your deeds realize the balance, or the lack of it, between your body's strength and your heart's love. Midway between the heart chakra and the third eye is the center in your throat, the center of your communications, of your words. Your words realize the balance, or the lack of it, between your heart's love and your mind's clarity. Your words and your deeds are the Ten Thousand that are born out of the three. All Ten Thousand, everything you have ever said or done, everything you are still proud of for the balance it has shown, or are still ashamed of for its lack, all Ten Thousand are a wall in front of you. However tall, however wide that wall, the next time you breathe out let it all slowly crumble and fall. Let all you have ever said or done settle and empty back into the Tao. As you breathe in, feel how balanced the Three can be. Let the Three settle and empty back into the Tao. And the Two and their dance. Let the Two dance their way back into the Tao. And the One, and all that light. Let everything settle and empty back into the Tao.

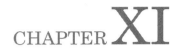

INTIMACY

Sex, Love, and Intimacy

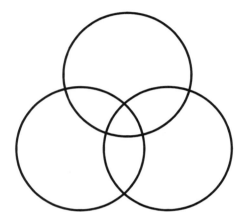

Confusion

Our confusion around sex, love, and intimacy, particularly our tendency to confuse sex and intimacy, underlies many of the problems we have in our relations with others, and seriously hampers our ability to become free in our bodies. There are occasions when two or all three of these are appropriately joined, and occasions when only one is present. This can be visualized as three intersecting circles with a rounded triangle in the center where all three join. Pointing out from each side of that center is an area where two circles intersect. The rest of each circle stands by itself. We need all three. In our lives we experience at one time or another every possible combination of these. Because we are multidimensional, rather than flat circles, these three are best visualized as intersecting spheres with which all the layers of our being, mind, body, heart, spirit, etc., interact. The layer of intimacy that is most often confused with sex is physical intimacy. We have a need for physical intimacy apart from sex that is often unacknowledged. This was our first need at birth, when we sought to re-establish physical contact with our mother. It is our need to be touched and held, and our need to touch and hold, for it is in the very nature of intimacy to break down the boundaries of doer and receiver, for both to just be, to be open, to be one at that point of contact.

Needs not met

Three ways this need can be thwarted or warped are- 1. By the inadequacy of our original bonding, by our not receiving the physical contact an infant requires. 2. By our being victims of abuse or incest. 3. By our education, our indoctrination in cultural attitudes that confuse sensuality with sexuality, and massage with prostitution, etc. A fourth factor might be the ways our seeking to fulfill that need have been rebuffed by others. The consequences of not fulfilling, of suppressing this need are far reaching. If we can not be intimate with our bodies we cannot be truly and fully intimate with any other part of our being. This does not mean we have to be physically intimate with everyone with whom we are emotionally or intellectually intimate. It means that if we are missing physical intimacy in our lives, all our other intimacies, including whatever spiritual intimacies we might have, have a hollow ring.

Physical intimacy   In our culture physical intimacy is more accepted between women than between men. For many men the only area where it is accepted is in contact sports. It's lack, and the hunger for it, underlie a common scenario in today's dysfunctional relationships-- when one party complains about their sexual needs, and the other about their emotional needs, not being met. Often the underlying unmet needs are for physical intimacy. When both parties understand and accept this need without confusing it with sex, the way is open for it to be met in each others' arms, and with others. Even in the most perfect marriage, at the center of which, love, sex and intimacy are beautifully integrated, non-sexual physical intimacy with others can enhance the relationship. Nurturing Bodywork such as Watsu and Tantsu, both receiving and giving, address directly this need, and help heal whatever wounds its non-fulfillment might have caused. In addition we can become more intimate with our own body, and get to know the energies moving through and around it, by stretching and practicing the movement meditations of this book. The ecstasy that moves our bodies when they become open, that vibrates, that undulates them in waves, should not be confused with sexual orgasm. It can happen when sex and intimacy are joined, and it can happen by itself when no sexual component is present. It is the orgasm of intimacy. Unlike a man's ejaculation or a woman's clitoral orgasm, it is not limited in space or time. There is no striving to reach it. There is no end, no separation, no before, no after.

Rapture   There is also an orgasm of love, a rapture, which can occur by itself, or in combination. When it occurs by itself, as in some forms of religious devotion, it is the very distance of the object of our love, its power, that fires us. When it occurs in combination with the ecstasy of intimacy, there can be no such separation because we are totally one with that object. This capacity for oneness is severely limited when our need for physical intimacy is denied and we are not free, not present, in our bodies.

On Becoming Intimate

Three elements   No matter on what level we become intimate, whether with another person or with our own body, with a place or with the world around us, there is a similar underlying process that entails three elements: 1. the knowledge of our separateness, 2. the opening to the other, and 3. the knowledge, the experience of our oneness. Any one of these can initiate the process, but there is no true intimacy unless all three are present. The delicacy of the balance between these three can be seen in our shifting relationship to our own body, at the extremes of which intimacy becomes impossible. At one extreme the separation is total and we look upon our body as object, a fearful object we are burdened with. At the other extreme, we are so totally one with its physicality that we lose sight of any part of our being that might not be limited to it. It is only between these extremes that true intimacy with our body becomes possible, when we are in our body and the oneness we feel is not limited by its physical boundaries. It is this middle ground, which Watsu is so effective at bringing us into.

Intimacy with place   Similar extremes and a middle ground appear in our intimacy with place. There are places we are out of place, and others that absorb us. Home is the middle ground. The intimacy that is home builds up over the years, but is not limited to one place. There are many places that are home. There are places we step into for the first time and have known all our lives, their completeness around us, a sacredness sending a shiver up our back. Intimacy can be that sudden.

Place in the world   There is a being at home in our body, and there is a place that is home, and there is our place in the world. When our lives unfold naturally without locking up in any one stage, we become more and more intimate with the world around us. The oneness of the newborn is not intimacy. It is before the knowledge of separateness. The first stage of development, the coming to terms with separateness, peaks in adolescence. The second is opening to the other. The third is coming into the oneness that is intimacy. The unfolding and interweaving of these three is punctuated by sudden intimacies, moments of enlightenment that reverberate throughout our lives. There is a stage before intimacy in the infant, and there is a final stage in the fully unfolded life, a coming home to the peace at the end, which is beyond intimacy.

Peace in the waves

A Watsu session can be a microcosm of our whole life and, like our life, it can be punctuated with moments of sudden intimacy, of waves that move our whole body. And there are moments of peace that are beyond intimacy. And there is peace in the waves.

Intimacy and Relationship

All three

This chapter opened with an exploration of how sex, love and intimacy are separate, overlapping, entities not to be confused. All three have their place in our lives: the intentionality of sex, the surrender of love and the oneness of intimacy. The more their separate natures are understood, the more we can experience how these three become one. Everything changes in a relationship in which sex, love and intimacy become one. Intimacies, ways of being intimate, levels of intimacy long hidden, open. The walls that society sets up between those levels fall. There is continuum in everything. Everything is sacred.

Relationships

As you develop in the work of this book, opening to the full range of intimacy, helping others in their opening to it, it is only natural that your relationships will evolve. As they do, whatever growth you experience in them will be reflected in your work. They are complementary.

Freedom and love

The freer you are in your own being the more you can be with others, the more you can be with one other. Freedom and love are not opposed. We can share the moment through time, extend it through the life of a relationship or marriage. Such a marriage is creation. Sharing the practices of this book, applying its principles on all levels, maintains that life, that creation, opens up all that intimacy has to offer.

A Marriage Manual

Be with your other in your freedom.
Love the freedom of your other
and all that it blossoms into.
Be flexible.
Be in the moment.
Be present.
Have no expectations.
Love is as shape-changing as water.
The still pond is beautiful.
The river rushing by is beautiful.
Waves wash up on the shore in ever new ways.
Water yields,
gives way,
surrounds whatever enters,
and allows it to move on through.
Hold like water.
Love like water.
When water is everywhere it has no goal.
Is the ocean here just to break on our shore?
And if it doesn't break is there no ocean?

CHAPTER XII

RESOURCES

This chapter explores some resources which can help make Watsu and its benefits available to more and more people. It ends with abbreviated notes of this book's sequences which can be photocopied and carried with you to sessions.

A Watsu Pool

There is finally an answer to the question so many of our Watsu students ask, "Where can I find a pool to watsu in?" The missing link in the development of Watsu has finally appeared in the form of a portable pool which is made specially for our students by one of the leading innovators in portable swimming pools. Its portability, and the ease with which it can be set up and taken down to store or transport or resell, makes it ideal for renters, and benefits homeowners as well by adding nothing to their property tax. It can be set up on any flat surface: yard, patio, basement or garage floor, etc. The pool can double as a spa or as an exercise pool for swimming in place. It can be seasonally moved outdoors and indoors. Practitioners can set it up at expos and fairs to help build a private practice at the same time they earn commissions selling pools, books and videos, etc. The pools will help bring Watsu into resorts, hotels, hospitals, clubs, chiropractor's offices, and in public, corporate and government fitness centers, etc.

Specifications

The pool is ten feet in diameter and holds four feet of water (almost 4000 gallons). It has a much longer life than pools with metal walls which rust, and liners which need regular replacement. Supported by snap together pvc pipes and fittings, the Watsu pool's single wall/liner is made of polytriply, an industrial strength polyester scrim (similar to what is used in radial tires), covered on both sides with a PVC coating. It is a little less thick than a nickel and has been treated for ultra violet light degradation and bacteria or fungus growth. The scrim has 20 high strength 100% polyester strands per vertical inch and 20 strands per horizontal inch, making it puncture resistant and impossible to tear. Its manufacturers, KD Pools, warranty the pool for five years.

Accessories

Insulating wrap around and floating blankets are available, as well as ozonaters and other equipment. A long time manufacturer of Geodesic domes has developed a kit for those who want to have a treated wood framework to cover, as needed, with material to keep rain or sun off and provide privacy.

If you are interested in obtaining and/or promoting this pool please contact the school (See page 125).

Where Watsu Began

Harbin Hot Springs

Some two hours north of San Francisco, Harbin Hot Springs, in whose pools Watsu was first developed, continues to be a resource for the continued growth of Watsu. Just as this place has nurtured the growth of Watsu, those who come and live here have found themselves nurtured in their growth by Watsu and the other forms of bodywork practiced here. The openness here is probably greater than at any other retreat or healing community in the world. Unlike Eselen in Big Sur, this place is open to the public 24 hours a day. The pools are always open.

Its growth

Twenty years ago the surviving structures of this century old resort were in ruins, their windows broken. But the springs never stopped flowing and the pools continued to attract a handful of people. One of them, Ishvara, purchased the springs and the 1100 acres around them which climb up to ridges on three sides, encompassing the whole valley Harbin is in. In order to set up a non-taxable community he formed the Heart Consciousness Church, a non-sectarian, non-guru church dedicated to the sanctity of each individual's path to spiritual growth, and deeded the property to it. He opened the doors to anyone who was respectful of the place and its people, and who wanted to help build it up as a workshop center. Today there are over 150 residents here working to maintain and develop further this beautiful, unique place. A second community has been started around another hot springs in the Sierras.

Coming to Harbin

People come from all over the world to enjoy Harbin's springs, the woods around, and the wide range of workshops presented here. I first came to soak in the springs and find people with whom I could practice the Zen Shiatsu I was studying. Later, when I started teaching Shiatsu, I regularly brought people up for workshops. I entered into partnership and eventually bought out a massage school that someone had brought here from Santa Cruz. The school has continued to grow and Harbin is now in the process of building us a center with our own pools on the side of Mt. Harbin.

The development of Watsu

In 1980 I began applying some of the stretches and moves of Zen Shiatsu while floating people in the warm pool here at Harbin. Over the subsequent years, with the help of students in countless classes here and in Europe, I gradually developed the Watsu featured in this book.

The community

Living here as a member of the Harbin community keeps me in contact with the way Watsu can effect a community, as well as visitors who come for sessions. Anyone coming here will find a book that lists several watsuers on staff here to choose from. You can come for the day, camp, or stay in a room. To get more information about Harbin Hot Springs and its community, or to reserve space in a dormitory or room, call (707) 987-2477 or fax (707) 987 0616.

How Watsu Spreads

Mainstream

One of our most valuable resources to help spread Watsu is the experience of others. Here, and at our International Watsu Conference held every November at a Hot Springs near Venice, watsuers come from all over to share their experiences. As would be expected, Watsu is finding its place in the mainstream therapy community. There are several fields, such as the treatment of abuse victims, where Watsu is becoming a therapy of choice. Its value to physical therapists is demonstrated in Chapter Seven. The subsequent chapter demonstrates how someone without physical problems can benefit from a series of sessions. Watsuers are successful here at Harbin and at other spas such as Two Bunch Palms in Desert Hot Springs and Ten Thousand Waves in Santa Fe. Its continued growth in the professional, the vertical, dimension is assured. Even more phenomenal is its growth in the horizontal direction, among non-professionals who benefit from sharing its simpler moves.

Ann Cole writes from Oregon, where she has been offering Watsu classes at an Easter Seal pool:

Watsu for Two

> When I returned from Harbin, I started the WATSU FOR TWO class out of my own experience of wanting to be able to give a Watsu to my husband and to all the people I love. I thought others would feel similarly. This class has run for almost a year now on a monthly basis and is the generator behind getting Watsu into the community. I give four one-hour classes teaching easy movements that anyone can do and then give each person an individual Watsu. I have had a paraplegic in my class, a woman who had a broken neck, a person with knee problems, people with fibromyalgia, arthritis, and chronic pain, mothers/daughters, lovers, friends, a rabbi, an acupuncturist, massage therapists, psychotherapists, physical therapists, recreational therapists, writers, a philosopher, a dancer, a brother/sister pair, a salesman, old and young, the whole unlikely cross section of humanity seems to have traveled through my class. It's wonderful! Then each week-one evening is set aside for people to give and receive basic Watsus with each other. People are beginning to make Watsu their own and are using it to heal themselves and their relationships.

Europe

In Europe Watsu is being used with a wide range of groups. In Montreaux it is a summer program offering for adolescents. The social services department in Geneva have sent seniors on retreats where they learn to watsu each other. In Italy childbirth trainers are teaching pregnant women, who are more comfortable in water than anyplace else, to watsu each other. They are also teaching husbands to Watsu their wives during pregnancy, and reporting how much it helps the husband sense and bond with his unborn infant. They also report that after delivery, it helps ease the tension that builds up in that period when the wife's interest in sex has not yet returned.

Family Therapy

In Germany, Monika Gurhoff finds that having people watsu each other helps deal with the wide range of physical and psychological problems that turn up in her Family Therapy practice. One case is a couple: The husband refuses to talk to the wife. The wife refuses sex. Watsu opens up for them an avenue of communication that is at once non-verbal and non-sexual, and brings them close again. In another case Watsu helps reform the bond between a mother and her hyper-active son. Monika also works with groups of women 60 to 80 years old whose childhood had been marred by the war and most of whom, being widows, only know physical contact in the context of painful medical operations. For these women, just holding and floating each other is a very profound experience.

Japan

The most recent example of Watsu's breadth, is how it is spreading in Japan. It is also an example of how one person in the right place can speed its spread. Two years ago, one of my students, Alice Kardon, introduced Watsu to a large group at an international conference on Water Exercise in Colorado. Among the participants was Jun Konno, the former head coach of the Japanese Olympic Swim Team. He had been introducing Water Exercise into Japan. Right away Jun saw Watsu as an ideal balance to those more aggressive exercises he had been learning in Europe and America, as something that could be used as a 'warm down' after a session. As he told me later, he also saw it as very appropriate for Japan, whose population is aging and becoming more isolated under the pressures of modern life. He ordered a video and book and began learning it. In the meantime, another student, Basia Szpak, told me she was taking a trip around the world to teach Watsu wherever she could. She was particularly interested in teaching it in Japan. I gave her Jun's address. After Israel, where Basia's Watsu made the front page, and Australia, where she had children watsuing each other and their parents, she arrived in Japan. Jun had organized two workshops for her with 150 people, most of them professionals in some form of aquatics, waiting to learn Watsu (and 9 assistants, who had learned from the video). It was very well received. The next summer Jun brought a group of aquatic exercise instructors here to Harbin to learn Watsu from me, something he plans to do every year. People all over Japan are concluding their Water Exercise sessions by taking each other in their arms and doing the Water Breath Dance.

Recent developments in Watsu have helped make it more accessible. Though I have not emphasized it in this book the way I did in my first, Watsu is a form of Bodywork Tantra. For me the essential ingredient of Tantra and Watsu is the absolute peace, the stillness, that is all the more powerful because it is at the center of all the movements of our energy. Over the years, rather than being a state to arrive at at the end of a Watsu, this stillness has come more and more to the forefront of Watsu. The recently developed Water Breath Dance is a beginning in stillness, a stillness that is returned to, that is maintained throughout a Watsu (which makes Watsu all the more Tantra). Besides helping people keep their movements as slow as their breath, its sinking and rising with a person is more of a being with them, and less of a 'doing' than the rocking I used to emphasize. Years ago when I first introduced the concept of the giver freeing his own body, I was thinking primarily of spontaneous movement. This is still true. Its waves do move us, but at the same time we find our freedom in the stillness. If there is no stillness, no movement is free. One result of Watsu's becoming stiller is that students are 'getting' Watsu much quicker and more easily. Watsu is becoming accessible to more people than it has ever been. The Watsu Round described below can bring large groups into this stillness in a short time. The Watsu Experience Weekend described afterwards gives people time to explore and experience this stillness before having to learn, to memorize moves.

The Watsu Round

For some time we have begun each intensive by having our students do the basic moves, rocking at least three other students in succession. An assistant would go up to the first student who has completed the basic moves with his first partner and take the recipient from the student, thereby freeing the student to take a partner from someone else, etc. This would continue until each student had the opportunity to do the basic moves with at least three people. What follows takes this process in a new direction, emphasizing sharing and being together rather than 'taking'. This is an ideal process to use with groups.

To start, divide participants into three groups: Givers, Receivers and Watchers. The last can be a smaller group than the first two. Givers do the Water breath dance with Receivers while Watchers stand to the side, each doing a solo water breath dance. When Giver feels completion in the open arm position he invites, with his eyes and his hands, a Watcher to join him on the other side of the Receiver. They do the Water breath Dance together holding Receiver between them. After bringing his knees to his chest with the breath (the accordion), they take Receiver to the wall, who stays there until he is ready to join the Watchers. Who had been Watcher becomes Giver and begins to watsu who had been Giver.

Before starting, an instructor needs to demonstrate the process and give instructions to each of the three groups.

Stand to the side, your feet spread and planted, and do the Water Breath Dance. Let your body sink to whatever direction it wants each time you breath out. Let the water bring you back up each time you breathe in. Watch those in the pool. Everyone is dancing. When someone invites you, move in close to the other side, the Receiver's left arm under your right arm. Slip your forearms under the Giver's and hold both elbows. Do nothing. Co-ordinate your breathing and sinking with the Giver. Let the Giver initiate the accordion and the taking of Receiver to the wall. Mirror every move from your side. After leaving Receiver at the wall, give to the one who had been Giver.

With Receiver's right arm behind your back, support the occiput with your left forearm and the tailbone with your right. Both hands are facing down. Start the Water Breath Dance, slowly sinking and rising to your own breath. Do not try to connect to the breathing of the person you are holding, but do keep the nose out of the water. Stay in this first position as long as it is comfortable. If your arm begins to tire, or if you feel complete in it, slide your arm under the knees and continue the Water breath Dance. When you feel complete in this second position, with your hands and eyes, invite a watcher you have not yet worked with to join you. Share, but do not make any effort to shift the person over to the watcher. Continue supporting and moving as before. When doing the Water Breath Dance together feels complete, begin letting the receiver's hips sink towards the bottom as the knees come closer to the chest with each outbreath. Open your arms and chest more and more each time you all three breathe in. Continue until this feels complete. Keeping the knees pressed to the chest, back the receiver up to the wall together. Temporarily supporting the near hip with your left knee, lower the foot to the ground. Once the back is straight against the wall, hold the near shoulder with one hand and the near hand with your other hand. Let go of the shoulder. Lift the hand towards the surface and back away. Stay still a moment. Receive.

Instructions to Receiver   As Receiver, do nothing. Just let your body go. Give feedback if anything is uncomfortable. When you feel the wall at your back, you'll know it has come to an end. Stay as long as you want at the wall. Then join the Watchers and do the Solo Water Breath Dance until someone invites you to join them.

Besides being an excellent introduction to Watsu, this round is a valuable process in its own right. It can be continued until everybody has had a chance to give to at least three different people.

Learning Watsu

The Watsu Experience Weekend   In teaching Watsu over the years, a recurrent problem has been how to teach students to become free and let go in their bodies on as deep a level as Watsu facilitates, and keep the sequence they are learning in mind at the same time. People who try to learn complicated sequences and moves too soon may miss the essential slowness, the grace of Watsu. We have recently developed the Watsu Experience to give people the opportunity to explore that slowness and experience that freedom thoroughly before having to focus on internalizing a sequence of moves. In a two day period they do the Watsu Round described above, and are shown and led into and out of all the positions of the Transition Flow. The emphasis is on just what it feels to be in each position, not on what comes next, to experience fully each position's potential for connection and letting go, both as receiver and giver. This makes a perfect weekend introduction to Watsu, which can be repeated over and over. If, in repeating these weekends and practicing, you master the Transition Flow, you would be eligible to enter our second level here at the school. The International Watsu Association described below, will provide instructors that can go anywhere to present this to any group that has facilities.

Trainings   Our trainings follow the structure outlined in this book. The first stage is to master the Water Breath Dance and the Transition Flow. Week long courses are regularly offered here at Harbin and in Europe. A second week expands the flow. A third week introduces further expansions and variations. Additional weeks focus on special uses of Watsu, and underwater work, etc.

Helping Watsu Spread

Building a clientele   There are many things you can do to help Watsu effect the lives of more and more people. Practicing and teaching are the most obvious. Our portable pool opens opportunities to demonstrate Watsu at gatherings such as the Whole Life Expo where exposure can help you build up a clientele. At the same time, if you wish to help market the pool, commissions would be available. Having local papers feature your work in articles can also help you build a practice. Offering Watsu to therapists, doctors and others in your community who might be able to refer clients is helpful. Find out what warm or warmable pools there are in your community. Volunteering their services at pools for the handicapped have helped some of our students get access to pools.

International Watsu Association   Our goal is to make everybody in the world a watsuer, to bring Watsu into as many lives as possible. The Association is not a union or closed shop. It is dedicated to making Watsu available. It provides instructors and information about where to find watsuers and pools. It publishes a newsletter which, in time, will grow into a regularly appearing journal.

Donations   Those who have the funds can help Watsu's become more widely available by donating to the Association, a non-profit corporation. Donations are urgently needed to finish the construction of a new Watsu Center here at Harbin, where, when we finally have our own pools, we will be able to train more watsuers and instructors and better explore the ways Watsu can realize its potential than is feasible in Harbin's more crowded pools. Besides deepening our trainings and focusing more on the special uses of Watsu (as with the handicapped, abuse victims and disturbed children etc.), we will explore how Watsu can assist and be integrated into a variety of personal growth processes. We will also explore various directions Watsu might open into, such as work underwater. Donations earmarked for developing a separate Watsu Center where its benefits could spread into your own community, are welcomed. We also welcome donations of labor and services. There is much, much work to be done, and many people whose lives could greatly benefit from this.

A Select Bibliography

Harold Dull, *Bodywork Tantra* (Harbin Springs, Middletown, 1987)
Shizuto Masunaga, *Zen Shiatsu* (Japan Press, New York, 1977)
Michel Odent, *Water and Sexuality* (Arkana, New York, 1990)
Burton Watson (Tr.), *Complete Works of Chuang Tzu* (Columbia, New York, 1968)
Kuang-Ming Wu, *The Butterfly as Companion* (SUNY, Albany, 1990)
Theodor Schwenk, *Sensitive Chaos* (Schocken Books, New York, 1976)
Elaine Morgan, *The Acquatic Ape* (Souvenir Press, London, 1982)
Deane Juhan, *Job's Body - A Handbook for Bodywork* (Station Hill, New York, 1987)
Margo Anand, *The Art of Sexual Ecstasy* (Tarcher, Los Angeles, 1989)

Videos

All of this book's sequences of Watsu and Tantsu are available on instructional videos. The Creative Movement Meditations are available on both video and audio tape.

For information about these, and the portable Watsu pool, as well as the latest dates and details about our trainings, write or call the school whose address is on the opposite page.

Pages to Copy

Many students have asked me for a simple explanation of Watsu that they could show others, so I am including the next page as a resource. Feel free to copy and use it in any way needed.

Following it are two pages of notes which may be copied and taken to the pool.

WATSU *Freeing the Body in Water*

To know what Watsu is, it must be experienced, if not in real water, at least in the imagination, which can be done because elements of Watsu have counterparts in everybody's experience.

Start with the way you relax when you lie back in warm water. Add how it feels to be stretched. Imagine how, in an element that removes pressure from joints and radiates warmth into muscle, you feel each stretch all the way through your body.

Add to the pleasure of being floated and stretched, what you feel in the best bodywork, when the tension in your neck is sensitively released, when your shoulder is rotated and freed, when just the right point is held. Imagine how that is amplified when, instead of weighing heavily on a table or floor, your body is free to move.

Add your most nurturing memory of someone holding, supporting you, just being with you, not trying to do something to you, holding you so lightly you feel your own lightness.

Combine all the above and there is still something to add- Watsu's flow. Watsu interweaves movement and stillness. It has a beginning and an end. And it is endless. Its lesson in letting go into the flow whatever comes up (and a lot does come up) can be carried into your everyday life. Its feeling of still being connected at the end when you're no longer being held can rebond you to that part of your being that is one with everything.

Now that you know what it is to receive a Watsu, the next step is to know what it is to give one. This too can be done in your imagination. Have you ever held a child sleeping in your arms? Have you ever danced with someone and felt the same music move both your bodies? Imagine floating someone level with your heart center, surrendering into the water each time you breathe out. Whatever direction you sink towards, the water lifts you back up as you breathe in. Imagine knowing a flow of moves in your body so well you are free to move to whatever waves of movement are created in each moment, waves that free both your bodies. Imagine coming to the end of a Watsu and lifting your hands off and still feeling connected.

Once you know what it is to give a Watsu, you will want to give it again and again, to discover each time, no matter how different each person is in your arms, that you are still one. Imagine how that knowing could set you free.

Imagine a world in which everyone watsued each other.

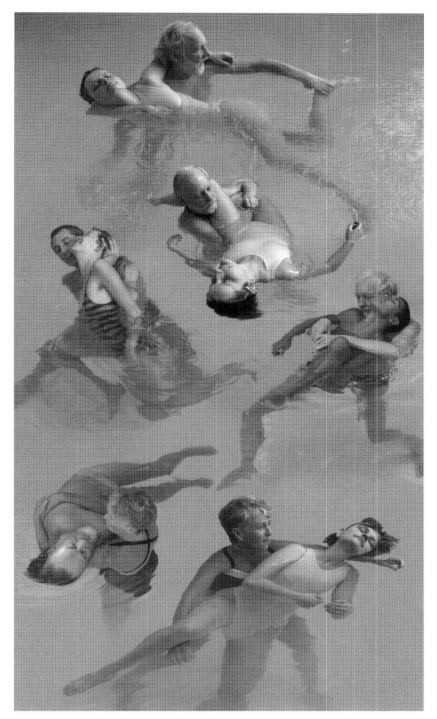

Watsu began when Harold Dull started floating people, applying the moves and stretches of the Zen Shiatsu he had studied in Japan. In the years since, Watsu has spread around the world and developed into a powerful form which professionals find alleviates a wide range of physical and emotional conditions. Everyone finds that sharing even Watsu's simplest moves can help free their bodies and enhance their sense of connection to others. For information about books, videos, classes (including instructors that could come to your pool), and a portable insulated Watsu pool write or call:

P. O. Box 570, Middletown CA 95461
Phone (707) 987 3801

SCHOOL OF SHIATSU & MASSAGE
HARBIN HOT SPRINGS

Basic Moves

a. Water Breath Dance	Begin from wall. Staying low in the water, feet spread, the neck in the crook of your left elbow, your right arm under the sacrum, the right arm behind your back, slowly sink and rise with your own breath.
b. Open Arms	Slide your right forearm under the knees. Balancing partner between your arms, continue to sink and rise.
c. Accordion	Sink partner deeper, gradually bringing the knees closer to the chest on each outbreath. Open arms on in-breath.
d. Rotating Accordion	Rotate both legs, bringing the knees close to the far shoulder on outbreath.
e. Near Leg Rotation	Rotating both legs, let the far leg slip off your forearm. Rotate near leg.

I Head Cradle

a. Capture	Sliding the head out your arm, hold the right knee from behind, turning partner just enough onto the side to draw the arm out from behind your back. Slip your right shoulder under the back of the neck.
b. Arm Leg Rock	Pull the left arm back with your left hand while your right holds the right leg back.
c. Twist	Pull the right knee across with your left hand while your right holds down the right shoulder.
d. Knee Head	Explore movement, the head in your right hand, the right knee in your left.
e. Second Side	Hold the left knee in your left hand and, making sure the left arm stays under yours, slip your left shoulder under the head. Work as above(b.-d.).
f. Stillness	Let partner float perfectly still, your right hand under the sacrum and your left under the head (Free Float).
g. Free Movement	Explore movement in this position.
h. Hip Rock	Lay the head on your left shoulder and move partner side to side, holding both hips. Return to position 1.

II Under Far Leg, Shoulder and Hip

a. Far Leg Over	After rotating near leg, rotate the far leg. Hold the foot in your right hand and wrap the leg around your neck.
b. Leg Push	Push the other leg away from you with your right hand while turning clockwise, your left hand pressing the upper back.
c. Sacrum Pull	Bending the knee, push the leg in front of you and around your waist. Hook the fingers of your right hand in the sacrum and pull.
d. Under Shoulder	Lay partner back and hold the float point under the back with your right hand as you slip out from under the left leg. Move under the shoulder with your right shoulder and place you right hand on the heart center.
e. Lengthening Spine	Push your left hand against the sacrum, lifting up as partner breathes in.
f. Spine Pull	Holding the occiput in your right hand, arm straight, move down to the left side, your left shoulder under the hip. Hook the fingers of your left hand into the top of the sacrum and pull to stretch spine.
g. Undulating Spine	Rhythmically lift left hand under sacrum to undulate spine. Hold float point with left hand and move into position 1 on left side.
h. Second Side	Do mirror image of a. - g. Repeat basic moves.

III Near Leg Cradle

a. Near Leg Over	Rotate near leg. Hold the foot in your right hand and wrap the leg around your neck.
b. Down Quads	Roll the muscles down the front of the far leg between fingertips and heel of your right hand.
c. Leg Down	Turning clockwise, push the left leg away from you and then, down against the inside of your right knee while swinging the torso up, the head against the knee. Pull the back while leaning into leg.
d. Leg Pass	Cross your left leg behind the left leg letting it float up toward surface.
e. Arm	Work arm with both hands. Pull left thigh to slip your shoulder out from under the right leg and return to position 1.
f. Second side	Do mirror image of a. - d.
g. Heart Home	Rock with your head on the heart. Rock with your right hand on the heart. Finish at wall.

I

a. Capture, b. Arm Leg Rock.

1. Arm Leg Rock II	Turn from side to side, maintaining pull of arm and leg.
2. Arm Opening	Free the left arm. Hold the hand and pull it up and back over the head, pulling the right knee at the same time.
3. Chest Opening	Hook your fingers into the upper corner of the chest. Pull back to stretch the chest open.
4. Shoulder Rotation	Hold firmly above shoulder joint and rotate left shoulder with your left hand.
5. Shoulder Blade	Lifting your thumb up between upper back and shoulder blade, work down inside of blade.
6. Bladder Meridian	Work down left of spine, rocking the body into your thumb. Hook left middle finger in point beside tailbone and rock.
7. Wall Knee	Lean back against wall. Pull right side of the lower back into your left knee, holding hara with left hand.

c. Twist, d. Knee Head Rock, e. Second Side, f. Stillness, g. Free Movement

8. Side Change	Move from side to side, pushing up against near hip at the same time as you pull the head and switch hands.

h. Hip Rock

9. Hara Rise	With right hand under the sacrum and your left on the hara, push down with the outbreath and up with the inbreath.
10. Buttock Rock	Hold a buttock in each hand as you move and rock partner.
11. Slide up Back	Brace your right hand against the top edge of the sacrum. Slowly slide your left hand lifting up the spine three times.
12. Forearm Lift	Holding the occiput and skull, alternately lift your forearms under the upper back.

II

a. Far Leg Over, b. Leg Push

1. Down Back	Hold upper back with left hand while right works down alongside spine. Hold point at top of leg and rock.
2. Foot	Bending and propping the leg across your hara, work foot.

c. Sacrum Pull, d. Under Shoulder, e. Lengthening Spine

3. Twist Over	Reach over near leg and pull up the left knee to twist stretch spine.
4. Figure Eight	Reaching under near leg, hold left foot and pull from side to side, inscribing the figure eight.
5. Lower Back	Press into the side of the lower back turned towards you with your forearm as you rock partner.

f. Spine Pull g. Undulating Spine

6. Thigh Rock	Clasp the left thigh tight to your waist and rhythmically tug.
7. Bow	Reaching under the near thigh, bracing the buttocks against your side, pull far leg back, arching the body.
8. Lift	Slip left arm under both knees. Swing partner up and brace on opposite hip. The head hanging forward, work the neck.
9. Neck Pull	Brace your left forearm against the top of the spine while pulling and working the neck with your right arm.

III

g. Second Side a. Near Leg Over, b. Down Quads

1. Up Liver	With the heel of your right hand, press the inside of the thigh up from the knee.
2. Down Bladder	Lifting with your thumb, work the midline down the back of thigh, knee and calf.

c. Leg Down, d. Leg Pass, e. Arm

3. Freeing the Arm	Squeeze, shake and move the opposite arm freely.

f. Second side, g. Heart Home

4. Hara Rock	Rock partner while holding and lightly squeezing the hara with your right hand.
5. Hara Spiral	While rocking partner work the meridian areas in the hara.

IVA

1. Leg Lift	Repeat the Basic Moves. While rotating the far leg, clamp the near leg between your thighs. Lift the far leg to stretch.
2. Hip Capture	Reaching under left leg, hold upper left arm and neck. Step between the legs and prop partner on your left hip.
3. Leg Tug	With your right arm hold the left thigh from underneath and tug.
4. Leg Rock	Leaning back against the right leg, rhythmically push the extended left leg out in front of you.
5. Leg Pull	Holding the occiput and the left foot stretch the whole body.
6. Foot Press	Holding the top of the left foot near the toes with your left hand, press the heel towards the left buttock.
7. Foot Prop	Prop the foot against the top of your leg (left if possible). Work right hand down bladder meridian. Work shoulder.
8. Face	Holding head in left hand, work face with right. Hold neck with both hands. Hold head in right; work face with left.
9. Second Leg	Reach under the right thigh and prop partner on your right hip to work mirror image of above (3 - 6).

IVB

1. Straddle	Back up to the wall and set partner straddling your left thigh, your left foot propped over your right knee.
2. Back Press	Both hands work down sides of spine pressing in with outbreath. Holding the last points beside the tailbone.
3. Up Back	Press fingertips into hip joints and make circular movements. Carry rapid circling on up back to behind left shoulder.
4. Shoulder Work	Work right shoulder. Slide scapula over your thumb on each outbreath work down scapula. Clasp and rotate shoulder.
5. Arm Back	Placing the arm behind the back. Hold upper arm with left hand while right squeezes down arm. Press palm into back.
6. Arm Rotation	Bracing the scapula with your right hand, rotate the arm.
7. Twist Across	Slip the arm between you. With right hand pull the wrist to your right side while your left pulls the left shoulder back.
8. Second Side	Move partner onto your right leg and do mirror image of above (4. - 7). Rest partner against your heart center a moment.
9. Uncradling	Start twisting partner to right. Before leg slips off pull knee to the chest with right hand. Pull both knees to the chest.

IVC

1. Knee Float	With the head on your left shoulder and a thigh in each hand, move partner about alternately rotating each leg..
2. Head Lift	Hold the occiput and skull in both hands and lift partner vertically. Set partner down on your left thigh.
3. Face Work	Lean your forehead against the back of the head and work the face with both hands
4. Chest Opening	Lay partner out close to the surface, tailbone on your left knee. Reaching under the arms, pull open the chest.
5. Heart-Hara	Hold partner, one hand on the heart center and the other on the hara.
6. Third Eye	Slide middle finger up nose to third eye. Raise both hands. Lift under palms with middle fingers. Float out to finish.

Afterword

There is no blue as blue as the sky is when you open your eyes floating on your back. This is the way to end a book. Floating. There is the freedom of movement, of flight. And there is the freedom of stillness. And the blue of the sky is that great bird Chuang Tzu saw the fish that is the dark of the northernmost sea rise up to become and fly over us on its way into the dark of the southernmost sea. It is a bird of a size that makes us tiny creatures floating below laugh. Laugh in waves, our bellies rising and falling with each breath. From dark to light to dark and back. And the ripples of our laughter spread across the surface, climb up onto the shore, and fly.

Chuang Tzu, you are our master of surprise and transformation. Your words weave every part of the void together with the joy and freedom of a body in water. And that butterfly you dream you are and wake up wondering if you are Chuang Tzu dreaming he is a butterfly or a butterfly dreaming he is Chuang Tzu, that butterfly is still fluttering among us watsuers, whispering "Keep it light. Keep it light. Keep it light."

note: Chuang Tzu and Lao Tzu (whose creation cycle is quoted earlier in this book) are founders of Taoism. Both Lao Tzu's laconic style, and the freedom of Chuang Tzu's writing, the way he joyfully, playfully draws in everything from the world around him, embody principles that centuries later will become the basis of Zen. The clearer we are, the more we are present to each moment, the more we are in touch with our participation in creation itself. Burton Watson's translation of Chuang Tzu's Inner Chapters has long been special to me. And now, just as I am finishing my book, a beautiful book on Chuang tzu's first three chapters, "The Butterfly as Companion" by Kuang-ming Wu, has come into my hands. The transmission is direct. The flow is uninterrupted from Taoism into Zen into Watsu. We all ride the same wave.